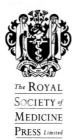

The ROYAL
SOCIETY of
MEDICINE
PRESS Limited

Atrial Fibrillation

in Practice

Gregory YH Lip

MD FRCP (Lond, Edin, Glasg) DFM FACC FESC
Consultant Cardiologist and Professor of
Cardiovascular Medicine, University
Department of Medicine, City Hospital,
Birmingham, UK

lymouth

Dedication

To my late parents, and those who suffer
from the most common of cardiac rhythm disorders

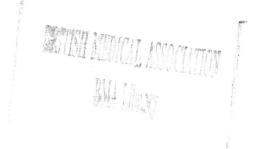

About the author

Gregory YH Lip MD FRCP (Lond Edin Glasg) DFM
FESC FACC is Professor of Cardiovascular
Medicine and Director of the Haemostasis,
Thrombosis and Vascular Biology Unit,
University Department of Medicine, City
Hospital, Birmingham. His research interests
range from clinical (atrial fibrillation,
hypertension, heart failure, ethnicity and
vascular disease, etc) to the laboratory
(thrombogenesis, atherogenesis and vascular
biology in cardiovascular disease and stroke).
He has published extensively on the clinical
epidemiology and pathophysiology of
thrombogenesis in atrial fibrillation, and the
use of antithrombotic therapy.

Preface

Atrial fibrillation is the most common cardiac rhythm disorder, but its management remains suboptimal. This book aims to address this deficiency by providing a clear, concise, management-orientated approach to atrial fibrillation, with the key points highlighted throughout the text, by boxes, tables and bullet points. Rather than provide a copious and detailed referenced text, references to the key papers have been made as 'Further Reading'. For greater detail, many comprehensive textbooks are available.

This book will hopefully provide a useful and practical guide to the issues relating to this common cardiac problem, to improve the care and treatment of these patients.

Gregory YH Lip
Birmingham 2001

Acknowledgements

Many colleagues and patients have kept my paroxysms of interest into atrial fibrillation persistent, to the extent that it is now permanent.

My gratitude also goes to Dr JW Mant and Dr R MacManus for an enlightening education into evidence-based atrial fibrillation which is evident in some sections of this book. I also thank Peter Altman of RSM Press, who persuaded me to complete the text, almost on schedule.

Contents

1. Epidemiology and importance

Introduction
Epidemiology
Incidence and prevalence
Clinical implications and importance
Does asymptomatic atrial fibrillation carry the same degree of risk as the symptomatic form?
Atrial fibrillation in the community
Atrial fibrillation in hospital practice
Atrial fibrillation and the patient

Introduction

Until fairly recently, atrial fibrillation (AF) was often regarded as an innocuous cardiac rhythm disorder, where patients could simply be treated with some digoxin and left well alone. Nothing could be further from the truth – AF is now recognized as a very important cause of mortality and substantial morbidity from heart failure, stroke and thromboembolism. Many patients with AF suffer from reduced exercise capacity as well as poor quality of life.

Indeed, AF is encountered in a wide variety of clinical settings. It may, for example, be discovered incidentally in an asymptomatic patient, it may develop in a patient who merely has a chest infection, fever or it may be found in a patient with a ventricular rate of 200 beats per minute who is too dizzy or lightheaded to stand up! While many are asymptomatic, many patients with AF have a wide variety of cardiorespiratory-presenting symptoms and clinical features, including syncope, heart failure

and stroke. Many patients may require long term treatment with potent antiarrhythmic and anticoagulant drugs, which may have important pharmacological interactions and adverse effects.

With the increasing age of the general population, AF is likely to become an even greater public health problem. Current perceptives of AF are summarized below.

Atrial fibrillation – the present
- Recent randomized controlled trials have clearly established the value of antithrombotic therapy in preventing stroke and thromboembolism in AF.
- Clinicians have recognized the limitations of simply treating AF with digoxin.
- Considerable advances have been made in the management of AF as more is understood about the underlying pathophysiology and electrophysiology of this condition.
- Better appreciation of the different clinical subtypes of AF, that is, paroxysmal (recurrent), persistent and permanent AF allows definition of objectives and strategies of management.

Epidemiology

The prevalence of AF varies widely around the world and varies according to the population studied. Much of the clinical epidemiology of AF is also based on data from predominantly Caucasian populations, and information on AF in non-Caucasian populations is scarce. Current perspectives on the epidemiology of AF are summarized below and in Table 1.1.

The risk of AF is well recognized to increase with age and with underlying heart disease. For example, the risk of AF has been found to be associated with increasing age, male sex, heart failure, valve disease, coronary heart disease, diabetes and hypertension. In the Cardiovascular Health Study, 57% of people with AF had clinical cardiovascular disease, and

Epidemiology of atrial fibrillation

- AF is the most common sustained cardiac rhythm disorder (Figure 1.1).
- AF is more common with increasing age, and is associated with common cardiovascular and non-cardiovascular diseases.
- Common cardiac causes of AF include hypertension, valve disease and ischaemic heart disease.
- Common non-cardiac causes of AF include thyroid disease, chest disease and intrathoracic pathology.
- Much of the clinical epidemiology of AF pertains to Caucasian populations. In Afro-Caribbeans, hypertension is likely to be the most common cause, while in Indo-Asians, ischaemic heart disease is the most common.

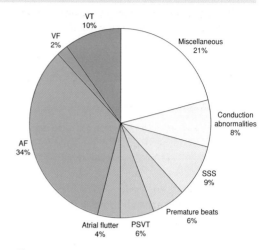

Figure 1.1
Hospitalizations for cardiac arrhythmias.
VT = ventricular tachycardia; VF = ventricular fibrillation; SSS = sick sinus syndrome; PSVT = paroxysmal supraventricular tachycardia; AF = atrial fibrillation. Adapted from Bialy *et al.* *J Am Coll Cardiol* 1992; **19**: 41A.

with AF had sub-clinical cardiovascular disease, and a further 35% had sub-clinical cardiovascular disease (being defined as abnormal findings on echocardiography or carotid ultrasound). Conversely, AF is uncommon in infants, children and healthy young adults.

Incidence and prevalence

The prevalence of AF approximately doubles with each advancing decade of age, from 0.5% at age 50–59 years to almost 9% at age 80–89 years (see Figure 1.2). AF is also becoming

Table 1.1
Ethnic differences in atrial fibrillation

	White (n=213)	Black (n=10)	Asian (n=22)
Age in years: mean (SD)	75.3 (11.0)	73.1 (12.1)	62.4 (15.5)
Past medical history			
None	19	1	2
Ischaemic heart disease	53 (24.9%)	1	10 (45/5%)
Valvular heart disease	11	0	2
Ischaemic and valvular heart disease	5	0	0
Thyroid disease	16 (7.5%)	0	0
Cardiomyopathy	0	0	2
Heart failure	39	3	4
Hypertension	45 (21.1%)	5 (50%)	1
Cerebrovascular disease	29 (13.6%)	0	2
Diabetes mellitus	22	0	2
Other	8	0	2

Adapted from Zarifis J *et al.* *Br J Clin Pract* 1997; **51**: 91–6.

significantly more prevalent, increasing in men aged 65–84 years from 3.2% in 1968-1970 to 9.1% in 1987–1989, an increase which is not explained by an increase in risk factors such as valve disease or myocardial infarction. It is estimated that more than one-half (56%) of people with AF are aged >75.

Applying age-specific prevalence rates to the population structure of England and Wales allows England and Wales specific estimates to be derived. Using this approach, the overall prevalence in England and Wales is 1.1%, rising to 6.1% in people aged >65, and to 8.6% in people aged >75.

AF is more common in men than women and over one-half (56%) of people with AF are aged >75. For example, in the largest UK study from Newcastle, the prevalence was 10% in men and 5.6% in women aged >75. Studies that have sub-divided AF into chronic and paroxysmal suggest that about one-quarter is paroxysmal, with the latter being younger and with a higher proportion (approximately 50%) being 'lone' AF.

In the Cardiovascular Health Study, the reported incidence for men aged 65 to 74 and 75 to 84 were 17.6 and 42.7 per 1000 person years respectively and for women, 10.1 and 21.6. Framingham study results were similar, but with smaller differences between men and women. On the basis of 38-year follow-up data from the Framingham Study, men had a 1.5-fold greater risk of developing AF than women after adjustment for age and predisposing conditions.

Clinical implications and importance

Key issues regarding the clinical implications and importance of AF are summarized in the box. The main burden of AF management rests with primary care clinicians as many do not present to hospital. Issues hence relate towards better detection and appropriate investigation of such patients.

Clinical implications and importance of AF

- AF represents a frequent problem not only for hospital physicians but also for primary care physicians.
- Most of AF appears to be managed by general practitioners, and in fact, only a third of patients with AF have ever been admitted to hospital.
- Surveys of AF in the community and among hospital admissions have consistently identified a sub-optimal application of standard investigations and treatment strategies, including a low rate of antithrombotic therapy (aspirin, warfarin) use and consideration of cardioversion to sinus rhythm.

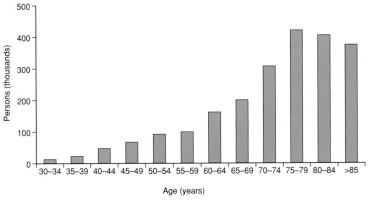

Figure 1.2
Estimated prevalence of AF in relation to age in the United States, based on four population-based surveys. The median age of AF patients is about 75 years. The overall number of men and women with AF is about equal, but approximately 60% of AF patients over age 75 years are female. Adapted from Feinberg WM, Blackshear JL, Laupacis A *et al*. Prevalence, age distribution, and gender of patients with atrial fibrillation: analysis and implications. *Arch Intern Med* 1995;**155**: 469–73.

In the Framingham study, over 40 years of follow-up, 621 people out of 5,209 developed AF, and this was associated with an adjusted 1.5 (men) to 1.9 (women)-fold increased risk of mortality. The median survival of people aged 55–64 in AF was 12.6 years for men and 12.1 years for women, as compared to 18.1 and 21.3 years respectively for those not in AF. Importantly, much of the mortality occurred early, often in the first 30 days of AF onset.

Stroke

The most common complication associated with AF is stroke, and indeed, there is a strong independent association between AF and stroke (Figure 1.3). When a patient with AF develops a stroke, the mortality is higher and there is a greater disability and lower discharge rate to their own home.

The proportion of strokes in the community that are attributable to AF rises with age. In the Framingham study, for example, AF was associated with 30.7% and accounted for 23.5% of strokes in people aged 80–89, compared with 8.5% and 2.8%, respectively, in those aged 60–69. The Oxford Community Stroke Project reported a higher 30-day case fatality rate for cerebral infarction associated

with AF (23%) as compared to those in sinus rhythm (8%). AF is associated with 30.7% and accounts for 23.5% of strokes in people aged 80–89, as compared to 8.5% and 2.8%, respectively, in 60–69 year olds. Another neurological complication associated with AF is impaired cognitive function and dementia (see below), which may in part be related to microemboli or ministrokes.

Coronary heart disease

Coronary heart disease is an important risk factor for the development of AF, and it is difficult to ascertain whether or not the excess risk of coronary heart disease in patients with AF represents a manifestation of pre-existing disease, or events attributable to AF. The prevalence of AF in uncomplicated coronary artery disease is also low, and much of the development of AF in these patients is often related to complications such as severe ischaemia or infarction and/or associated heart failure.

However, in the Framingham study, it appears that the mortality from coronary heart disease is three-fold higher (6.4% vs 1.7%) for men in general, but particularly for men with AF (3.1% vs 0.8%) compared with matched controls in sinus rhythm.

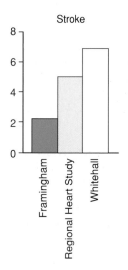

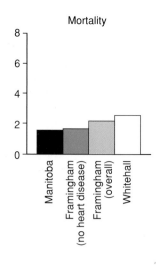

Figure 1.3
Relative risk of stroke and mortality in patients with AF compared with patients without AF. Source data from the Framingham Heart Study, British Regional Heart Study, Whitehall study, and Manitoba study.
Reproduced with permission from Fuster V *et al.* *J Am Coll Cardiol* 2001; **38**:1231–65. Copyright 2001 by the American College of Cardiology and the American Heart Association, Inc.

Heart failure

Heart failure associated with AF has a worse prognosis than heart failure without AF, although this is likely to be improving, in the light of improvements in heart failure management and avoidance of Class Ia antiarrhythmic agents, such as quinidine, disopyramide and procainamide. For example, the prognosis for heart failure in association with AF improved from a two-year survival of 39% between 1985–1989, to 66% between 1990–1993. An important retrospective analysis from the SOLVD (Studies Of Left Ventricular Dysfunction) studies reported that patients with AF had greater all-cause mortality (34% vs 23%, $p<0.001$), death attributed to pump failure (16.7% vs 9.4%, $p<0.001$) and were more likely to have the endpoint of 'death or rehospitalization for heart failure' (45% vs 33%, $p<0.001$), when compared with those in sinus rhythm. However, there was no difference in deaths caused by cardiac arrhythmias. The presence of heart failure also increases the risk of stroke and thromboembolism in AF, and the presence of moderate to severe left ventricular dysfunction on 2-dimensional echocardiography is an independent risk factor for stroke on mutivariate analysis.

Cognition/dementia

There is a recognized association between AF and poor cognitive function. Interestingly, the association with AF was with Alzheimer's disease rather than vascular dementia. In a survey of 952 men aged 69–75 in Sweden, lower scores on cognitive function tests were attained by the 44 men in AF as compared to those in sinus rhythm, after adjusting for age, blood pressure, diabetes and ejection fraction.

In the Rotterdam study, AF was associated with both cognitive impairment and with dementia, after a 'dementia work up' (cognitive function tests, through to detailed neuropsychological testing and brain magnetic resonance imaging [MRI] where indicated).

Does asymptomatic atrial fibrillation carry the same degree of risk as the symptomatic form?

Most patients (90%) referred to outpatients who are found to be in AF have symptoms. The prevalence of asymptomatic AF in the community is unknown. In the Newcastle survey, 71 of 93 (76%) patients found to be in AF were already known to their general practitioner. The remainder (24%) may offer a crude proxy for asymptomatic AF in the community.

However, there is no evidence as to whether or not the risk of asymptomatic AF conferred a better prognosis or otherwise. Indeed, this factor was not used as a clinical variable in analyses of clinical risk factors of thromboembolic risk in various meta-analyses. However, given that some of the independent clinical predictors of thromboembolism are themselves associated with symptoms (eg heart failure, previous stroke), it is likely that asymptomatic AF could possibly be associated with lower risk.

Atrial fibrillation in the community

The general practitioner is likely to remain as the 'front line' for the initial detection, assessment and management of patients with AF. Certain patient categories should be referred for specialist assessment.

Role of the general practitioner

- Most general practitioners manage AF and few affected individuals are admitted to hospital.
- The GP is important in identification of patients with new onset AF.
- Most GPs can assess thromboembolic risk and facilitate the early initiation and monitoring of antithrombotic therapy.
- GPs should refer appropriate patients to a cardiologist for further assessment (including echocardiography) and consideration of cardioversion.
- GPs should be aware of potential drug interactions and toxicity with antiarrhythmic drugs and anticoagulants.

When to refer a patient with AF to a cardiologist

- Patient aged below 30 years
- AF resistant to 'usual' drugs for rate control
- Patient suitable for cardioversion (see chapter 8)
- Further assessment required, eg valvular heart disease
- Patient with moderate to severe heart failure
- Patient with resistant heart failure
- Frequent attacks of paroxysmal AF
- Syncopal attacks due to AF

presence of an irregular pulse, will require further investigation with an ECG. It is thus important to know when to 'screen' for AF among the patients attending for a general practice consultation.

When to screen for AF in general practice

- Patient complaining of palpitations or syncope
- Patient with stroke or transient ischaemic attacks
- Patient with heart failure
- Patient on regular diuretic or digoxin therapy

Individuals who are at 'high risk' of developing AF, such as those with hypertension, heart failure, thyroid disease or ischaemic heart disease, should be screened for AF. For example, AF is present in approximately one-third of patients with heart failure, while subclinical hyperthyroidism is common in the elderly who may not exhibit overt symptoms of the latter condition.

Recent onset symptoms of palpitations or reduced exercise tolerance, especially in the

Anticoagulation and the general practitioner

Despite the compelling evidence of the benefits of stroke reduction in patients with AF, antithrombotic therapy continues to be suboptimal, ranging from 11% to 44% in those eligible for oral anticoagulants. How to deliver anticoagulation therapy is an important consideration.

Table 1.2

Attitudes of GPs and hospital consultants on anticoagulant therapy in general practice

Consultants	GPs		Hospital	
	Agree	Disagree	Agree	Disagree
More management of warfarin anticoagulation should be undertaken in primary care	43%	18%	58%	17%
Patients would prefer to have their warfarin anticoagulation managed by their GP	60%	6%	43%	8%
GPs cannot initiate warfarin anticoagulation as efficiently as hospital provided services	32%	42%	40%	38%
GPs cannot monitor warfarin anticoagulation as efficiently as hospital provided services	21%	62%	28%	50%
GPs do not have enough experience to manage the warfarin anticoagulation of their patients	18%	60%	27%	37%
Warfarin anticoagulation treatment can be safely initiated by GPs	56%	19%	61%	22%
Warfarin anticoagulation treatment can be safely monitored by GPs	87%	5%	77%	12%

Adapted from Rodgers H, Sudlow M, Dobson R et al. Br J Gen Pract 1997; **47**: 309–10.

Many health authorities and general practitioner groups have attempted to address this by providing guidelines for the use of anticoagulation in AF. It has been estimated that if various guidelines were applied to a hypothetical population of patients with AF, the rate of anticoagulation would range from 13% to 100%.

One suggested option to improve anticoagulation management of these patients with AF may be to increase involvement of general practitioners. Although regular monitoring of anticoagulation intensity and adjustment of dosage is often done at hospital- or satellite-community-based anticoagulant clinics, some general practitioners now undertake this task. Many general practitioners do feel they can take on this role, given appropriate training, resource and support.

If better, safer and increasing use of anticoagulation in patients with AF is intended, increasing provision of general practitioner-based anticoagulation monitoring aided by computerized support system and near patient testing may become a necessary step.

Indeed, anticoagulant monitoring by general practitioners has been found to be much better than that in hospital clinics. Furthermore, many patients prefer to attend their local general practitioner rather than busy hospital clinics which may be far away. However, there is some variation in the willingness and ability of general practitioners to undertake anticoagulation monitoring (Table 1.2).

Screening for atrial fibrillation

Screening for AF would result in an increasing referral rate for specialist advice and cardiological investigations (such as echocardiography). A screening programme for AF in general practice would result in the requirement for 625 echocardiographic examinations in each district general hospital serving a population of 250,000; this might potentially prevent 19 strokes in each year. Open access to general practitioners for echocardiography in local hospitals for patients with heart failure has been tried successfully in some centres and there is a good case for extending this facility to the management of AF. There are still some unresolved questions over screening for AF.

The simplest screening strategy for AF is one of an 'opportunistic case finding' programme, where a general practitioner will feel a patient's pulse during a consultation; if abnormal, an electrocardiogram (ECG) would be performed as a confirmatory test. However, opportunistic case finding is likely to miss many people who would otherwise have benefited from treatment, especially the majority of AF patients in the community who may be asymptomatic or those with paroxysmal AF, who happen to be in sinus rhythm at time of checking the pulse. In the Newcastle survey, the sensitivity of pulse palpation was 93–100%, and specificity 71–86%, with lower values in the elderly. Little advantage was found by adding the prescription of digoxin as an additional screening tool. While the irregularity of the pulse in AF is classic teaching, up to one-third of cases may have regularity of rhythm and >50% of cases have regularity of pulse volume.

Another possible approach is to screen patients at higher risk of AF – a 'targeted screening' programme. For example, heart failure, myocardial infarction, diabetes, hypertension and rheumatic heart disease are important precursors of AF, as well as those with a history of hyperthyroidism, stroke or transient ischaemic attack. A third possible approach is to screen everyone over the age of 65 years for AF – a 'whole population' screening programme, which would have significant implications for resources and costs.

Atrial fibrillation in hospital practice

As with general practice, the increasing prevalence of AF anticipated for the future will mean there will be more patients at increased risk of stroke and heart failure, with a significant mortality and morbidity. The increasing prevalence and incidence of AF is likely to impact on provision of investigations such as echocardiography, 24-hour Holter monitoring.

The increasing use of warfarin for thromboprophylaxis also requires regular attendances at a hospital anticoagulant clinic for monitoring of the International Normalised Ratio (INR). If such patients are reliant on expensive hospital-provided transport, this adds to the overall costs of treating such patients, and one option is to run domiciliary anticoagulant checks, which minimize this expense.

Postoperative AF is also a healthcare problem. For example, AF after cardiac surgery can occur in approximately one-third of patients and is associated with an increase in adverse events in all measurable outcomes of care and increases the use of hospital resources and, therefore, the cost of care.

Atrial fibrillation and the patient

Many patients with AF possess limited knowledge of AF as well as its consequences and therapy. Furthermore, we have recently highlighted significant differences between different ethnic groups in terms of their knowledge of the risks, actions and benefits of warfarin as well as AF itself.

In our survey of 119 patients with AF (33% of whom were Indo-Asian, 23% Caribbean and 44% Caucasian), only 63% of the overall study cohort was aware of their cardiac condition, with Indo-Asians and AfroCaribbeans significantly less aware of AF compared to the Caucasian patients. When questioned about the perception of the severity of the underlying condition, the majority of patients (61%) felt that AF was 'not serious', and a large proportion were unaware that AF predisposed to thrombosis and stroke. Only 52% in the whole cohort were aware of the reason(s) for commencing their warfarin while the remainder commenced warfarin simply because 'doctor told them so'. Many patients with AF also felt that their doctor had not given them enough information about their warfarin therapy. Patient understanding and education and active participation in their management are therefore important to ensure an holistic approach to AF management.

Further reading

Benjamin EJ, Levy D, Varizi SM et al. Independent risk factors for atrial fibrillation in a population based cohort: the Framingham Heart Study. JAMA 1994; **271:** 840–4.

Benjamin EJ, Wolf PA, D'Agostino RB et al. Impact of atrial fibrillation on the risk of death: the Framingham Heart Study. Circulation 1998; **98:** 946–52.

Brand FN, Abbott RD, Kannel WB, Wolf PA. Characteristics and prognosis of lone atrial fibrillation: 30-year follow-up in the Framingham Study. JAMA 1985; **254:** 3449–53.

Dries SL et al. Atrial fibrillation is associated with an

increased risk for mortality and heart failure progression in patients with asymptomatic and symptomatic left ventricular systolic dysfunction – a retrospective analysis of the SOLVD trials. *J Am Coll Cardiol* 1998; **32**: 695–701.

Feinberg WM, Blackshear JL, Laupacis A *et al*. Prevalence, age distribution and gender of patients with atrial fibrillation. *Arch Intern Med* 1995; **155**: 469–73.

Furberg CD, Psaty BM, Manolio TA *et al*. Prevalence of atrial fibrillation in elderly subjects (the Cardiovascular Health Study). *Am J Cardiol* 1994; **74**: 236–41.

Kannel WB, Wolf PA, Benjamin EJ, Levy D. Prevalence, incidence, prognosis and predisposing conditions for atrial fibrillation: population-based estimates. *Am J Cardiol* 1998 Oct 16; **82**(8A): 2N–9N.

Kilander L, Andren B, Nyman H *et al*. Atrial fibrillation is an independent determinant of low cognitive function. A cross sectional study in elderly men. *Stroke* 1998; **29**: 1816–20.

Kopecky SL, Gersh BJ, McGoon MD *et al*. Lone atrial fibrillation in elderly persons: a marker for cardiovascular risk. *Arch Intern Med* 1999; **159**: 1118–22.

Lake FR, Cullen KJ, de Klerk NH *et al*. Atrial fibrillation and mortality in an elderly population. *Aust NZ J Med* 1989; **19**: 321–6.

Levy S, Maarek M, Coumel P *et al*. A Characterization of different subsets of atrial fibrillation in general practice in France: the ALFA study. *Circulation* 1999 Jun 15; **99**(23): 3028–35.

Lin H-J, Wolf PA, Kelly-Hayes *et al*. Stroke severity in atrial fibrillation. *Stroke* 1996; **27**: 1760–4.

Lip GYH, Bawden L, Hodson R. Atrial fibrillation among the Indo-Asian general practice population. The West Birmingham Atrial Fibrillation Project. *Int J Cardiol* 1998; **65**: 187–92.

Lip GYH, Golding DJ, Nazir M *et al*. A survey of atrial fibrillation in general practice: The West Birmingham Atrial Fibrillation Project. *Br J Gen Pract* 1997; **47**: 285–9.

Lip GYH, Tean KN, Dunn FG. Treatment of atrial fibrillation in a district general hospital. *Br Heart J* 1994; **71**: 92–5.

Lip GYH, Zarifis J, Watson RD, Beevers DG. Physician variation in the management of patients with atrial fibrillation. *Heart* 1996; **7**: 200–5.

Lip GYH, Kamath S, Jafri M, *et al*. Ethnic differences in patient perceptions of atrial fibrillation and anticoagulant therapy. The West Birmingham Atrial Fibrillation Project. *Stroke* 2001; (in press).

O'Connell J, Gray CS. Atrial fibrillation and stroke prevention in the community. *Age Ageing* 1996; **25**: 307–9.

Office for National Statistics. 1998 mortality statistics – cause. Series DH2 no. 25. London: The Stationery Office, 1999.

Ott A, Breteler M, de Bruyne MC *et al*. Atrial fibrillation and dementia in a population based study. *Stroke* 1997; **28**: 316–21.

Psaty BM, Manolia TA, Kuller LH *et al*. Incidence of and risk factors for atrial fibrillation in older adults. *Circulation* 1997; **96**: 2455–61.

Rawles JM. What is meant by a 'controlled' ventricular rate in AF? *Br Heart J* 1990; **63**: 157–61.

Sandercock P, Bamford J, Dennis M *et al*. Atrial fibrillation and stroke: prevalence in different types of stroke and influence on early and long-term prognosis (Oxfordshire Community Stroke Project). *BMJ* 1992; **305**: 1460–5.

Stevenson WG *et al*. Improving survival for patients with AF and advanced heart failure. *J Am Coll Cardiol* 1996; **28**: 1458–63.

Sudlow M, Rodgers H, Kenny RA, Thomson RG. Service provision and use of anticoagulants in atrial fibrillation. *BMJ* 1995; **311**: 558–61.

Sudlow M, Rodgers H, Kenny RA *et al*. Population based study of use of anticoagulants among patients with atrial fibrillation in the community. *BMJ* 1997; **314**:1529–30.

Sudlow M, Thomson R, Thwaites B *et al*. Prevalence of atrial fibrillation and eligibility for anticoagulants in the community. *Lancet* 1998; **352**: 1167–71.

Wheeldon NM, Tayler DI, Anagnostou E *et al*. Screening for atrial fibrillation in primary care. *Heart* 1998; **79**: 50–5.

Wolf PA, Abbott RD, Kannel WB. Atrial fibrillation as an independent risk factor for stroke: the Framingham study. *Stroke* 1991; **22**: 983–8.

Wolf PA, Abbott RD, Kannel WB. Atrial fibrillation: a major contributor to stroke in the elderly. The Framingham Study. *Arch Intern Med* 1987; **147**: 1561–4.

Zarifis J, Beevers DG, Lip GYH. Acute admissions with atrial fibrillation in a British multiracial hospital population. *Br J Clin Pract* 1997; **51**: 91–6.

2. Aetiology

Hypertension
Coronary artery disease
Heart failure
Valve disease
Congenital heart disease
Cardiomyopathy and pericardial
disease
Alcohol
Thyroid disease
Chest disease
Familial atrial fibrillation
Lone atrial fibrillation

Common causes of atrial fibrillation

Cardiovascular causes	Noncardiovascular causes
Hypertension	Hypoxia and respiratory failure
Coronary artery disease	Diabetes
Cardiomyopathy	Drugs (cocaine, theophylline, alcohol, caffeine)
Mitral valve disease	Hyperthyroidism
Pericarditis	Postoperative thoracotomy
	Electrolyte abnormalities (low K^+ and Mg^{2+}, high Ca^{2+})

Hypertension

In developed countries, hypertensive heart disease is currently the most common underlying disorder in patients with atrial fibrillation (AF). In the Framingham study, hypertension was considered to be the most common cause of AF, being present in over 50% of subjects. The presence of hypertension was associated with a relative risk of 1.9 for developing AF, and may be the most common underlying cause in black or Afro-Caribbean patients.

AF and hypertension

- Chronic hypertension, with associated left ventricular hypertrophy and/or diastolic dysfunction, results in an increase in left atrial pressure and left atrial dilatation.
- The latter alters the electrophysiological properties of the atrium resulting in the propensity to develop AF.
- Excess alcohol intake may contribute to both hypertension and AF.
- Patients with hypertension are more prone to developing coronary artery disease, which is another important risk for developing AF.
- Hypertension is additive to the risk of stroke and thromboembolism in AF.

Coronary artery disease

There is a high prevalence of coronary artery disease (CAD) in the population, and thus CAD is commonly stated as a frequent cause of AF. AF is not, however, commonly associated with isolated CAD *per se*, unless these patients are 'complicated' by sustaining a myocardial infarction or have underlying heart failure. AF in the setting of chronic angina is usually associated with left ventricular impairment, especially diastolic dysfunction, as a result of ischaemic heart disease.

Postoperative AF contributes to significant morbidity, increased length of hospital stay, and increased costs in cardiac surgical patients. AF occurs in 40% of coronary artery bypass graft patients and 60% of those undergoing valve surgery. The frequency of AF peaks on day 2–3 post surgery. Prophylaxis of AF with beta-blocker therapy is an effective treatment strategy while digoxin and verapamil are ineffective.

AF and coronary artery disease

- Uncomplicated coronary artery disease is an uncommon cause of AF.
- AF frequently develops in association with 'complicated' coronary artery disease, such as myocardial infarction or heart failure.
- AF may develop during acute myocardial infarction, where it is usually transient (in the first 24 hours), but may be associated with increased mortality, larger infarcts, heart failure and thromboembolism.
- AF following coronary artery bypass surgery is common (25–30%) and is an important cause of morbidity and prolonged hospital stays.
- Fast AF may result in angina due to the rapid ventricular response.

Predictors of postoperative AF

- Prior AF
- Age greater than 60 years
- Valve surgery
- History of heart failure
- Preoperative beta-blocker therapy (probably with abrupt withdrawal)
- Intraoperative techniques (debated)
- Hypokalaemia

Heart failure

AF occurs frequently in association with heart failure, and the presence of the latter can result in significant haemodynamic disturbance as well as an increase in the risk of stroke and thromboembolism. Approximately one-third of patients with heart failure have AF, although this proportion is higher in more severe cases. Conversely, left ventricular dysfunction is present in approximately one-third of patients with AF.

A study in Hillingdon, west London, found a population incidence of heart failure of 1.3 cases per 1000 population per year for those aged >25. Of these, AF alone was thought to be the primary aetiology in 5% of 220 patients. Wheeldon et al studied patients with AF in primary care (65 patients aged >65) and found that symptoms suggestive of cardiac failure were common (32%), and echocardiography identified co-existing cardiac problems, the most common being left atrial dilation (80%), mitral regurgitation (48%), mitral annular calcification (43%) and left ventricular hypertrophy (32%).

AF can predispose to heart failure by causing fast ventricular rates and rate-related ischaemia; and congestive heart failure can lead to AF due to high intracardiac pressures. As AF can cause heart failure and *vice versa*, this leads to a 'chicken or egg' situation when evaluating a patient with AF and heart failure. Furthermore, uncontrolled fast AF rates can lead to left ventricular dilatation and systolic impairment, the so-called 'tachycardia-induced cardiomyopathy' or 'tachycardiomyopathy' with electromechanical feedback and neurohumeral activation playing a role. Alcohol can be an important precipitant of AF and chronic alcohol use can result in heart failure due to alcoholic cardiomyopathy. Finally, both AF and heart failure are closely related to heart disease and hypertension.

Valve disease

Rheumatic heart disease is infrequent in developed countries, but worldwide, rheumatic valve disease is still an important cause of AF. While AF is usually associated with mitral stenosis or mitral regurgitation, AF can also occur in association with aortic stenosis, where it can result in heart failure and haemodynamic deterioration.

Valve disease is particularly important since mitral valve disease increases the thromboembolic risk of patients with chronic AF by approximately 18-fold. Up to 20% of patients with mitral stenosis and AF develop embolic events and these most commonly (60–75%) affect the cerebral circulation. This risk of stroke and thromboembolism for patients in AF is three to seven times greater than in patients with mitral stenosis in sinus rhythm.

Congenital heart disease

AF can be associated with congenital heart disease, especially atrial septal defect and Eisenmenger's syndrome. As many such patients are now surviving to adulthood, the development of AF may result in clinical deterioration or cardiac decompensation, as well as the need for antithrombotic therapy.

Cardiomyopathy and pericardial disease

The development of AF in patients with hypertrophic cardiomyopathy, who are likely to have diastolic dysfunction, may result in haemodynamic compromise. Any pericardial disease can cause AF. Less common causes of AF include peripartum cardiomyopathy, lupus myocarditis, the cardiomyopathy associated with severe obesity and both idiopathic and uraemic pericarditis.

Alcohol

Cardiac arrhythmias, especially supraventricular arrhythmias, occur more frequently in heavy alcohol drinkers, particularly after a weekend or holiday-related bouts of heavy consumption. In one Scandinavian series, alcohol caused or contributed to new onset AF in young subjects in 63% of cases, hence the term 'holiday heart syndrome', referring to acute disturbances of cardiac rhythm with heavy alcohol consumption in people with 'normal hearts'. In younger patients (aged <65 years) with new onset AF, alcohol intake should be questioned.

Thyroid disease

Thyroid disease may be an underdiagnosed cause of AF, as thyroid function tests are often neglected, particular in the elderly in whom classic signs of thyrotoxicosis may not be obvious.

Krahn et al reported that of 726 patients with recent onset (<3 months) AF, only five (0.7%) were hyperthyroid (TSH<0.1 mU/l) and none was hypothyroid. This would suggest a low

---

Mechanisms for alcohol-related AF

- Increases in levels of catecholamines during acute alcohol ingestion.
- The direct toxic effect of alcohol exerted by acetaldyhyde on the myocardium and changes in conduction and refractory times.
- Alcohol may also cause arrhythmogenic changes in serum electrolyte concentrations.
- Acute alcohol ingestion can influence the parasympathetic system, especially with vomiting; such vagal stimulation can provoke atrial arrhythmias.
- Alcohol use is related to hypertension, which is an important cause of AF.
- Alcohol may result in a dilated cardiomyopathy-like picture, resulting in high intra-atrial pressures and the development of AF.

---

yield for picking up associated thyroid disease, although it should be appreciated that thyroid disease is very much a treatable cause of AF. One clinical clue to underlying thyrotoxicosis may be the failure of digoxin to control the ventricular rate without the addition of beta-blockers.

Attempted electrical or pharmacological cardioversion should not be attempted while the patient remains thyrotoxic, as AF usually recurs if the hyperthyroidism remains uncontrolled. Spontaneous reversion to sinus rhythm often occurs in six weeks in younger patients who are rendered euthyroid; older patients show less spontaneous reversion. A summary of AF and the thyroid is shown.

Chest disease

Acute and chronic pulmonary or pulmonary-vascular disease such as pneumonia, acute pulmonary embolism and chronic obstructive pulmonary disease may all present with AF. In fact, any thoracic pathology can cause AF – this can range from a simple pyrexial infection to lung carcinoma, pericardial disease, infections and pleural disease. Up to 10% of patients with documented pulmonary

---

AF and thyroid disease

- AF occurs in about 20–25% of older patients with thyrotoxicosis, but is uncommon under the age of 30.
- Thyroid function tests should always be checked in a patient newly presenting with AF.
- In the elderly, thyroid disease may be subclinical.
- Increased beta-adrenergic tone may be in part responsible for the development of AF and may also contribute to the rapid ventricular response in this disorder.
- Cardioversion should not be attempted until the thyroid disorder is treated.

---

thromboembolism have AF, although the most common ECG abnormality in this condition remains sinus tachycardia.

Familial atrial fibrillation

In 1997, Brugada *et al* described a family of 26 members of whom 10 had familial AF, the condition segregated as an autosomal dominant trait. Genetic linkage analysis has localized the responsible gene to chromosome 10q in the region of 10q22–q24, which may contribute to the substrate for the development of AF.

Lone atrial fibrillation

This is a diagnosis of exclusion where heart disease and other precipitating causes of AF have been excluded by careful history and clinical examination. Furthermore, these patients should have a normal 12-lead ECG (apart from the AF), normal chest X-ray and a structurally normal heart on echocardiography. Different studies have used slightly different diagnostic criteria for lone AF, but in general, about 20% of sustained AF is 'lone AF', compared to approximately 50% of paroxysmal

AF being 'lone AF'. Strictly defined lone AF in young individuals (age <65 years) is associated with a low thromboembolic risk, and antithrombotic therapy may not be required.

Further reading

Atrial Fibrillation Investigators. Echocardiographic predictors of stroke in patients with atrial fibrillation: A prospective study of 1066 patients from three clinical trials. *Arch Intern Med* 1998; **158**: 1316–20.

Benjamin EJ, Levy D, Varizi SM *et al*. Independent risk factors for atrial fibrillation in a population based cohort: the Framingham Heart Study. *JAMA* 1994; **271**: 840–4.

Brand FN, Abbott RD, Kannel WB, Wolf PA. Characteristics and prognosis of lone atrial fibrillation: 30 year follow-up in the Framingham study. *JAMA* 1985; **254**: 3449.

Brugada R, Tapscott T, Czernuszewicz G *et al*. Identification of a genetic locus for familial atrial fibrillation. *N Engl J Med* 1997; **336**: 905.

Cowie MR, Wood DA, Coats AJ *et al*. Incidence and aetiology of heart failure; a population-based study. *Eur Heart J* 1999 Mar; **20**(6): 421–8.

Dries DL, Exner DV, Gersh BJ *et al*. Atrial fibrillation is associated with an increased risk for mortality and heart failure progression in patients with asymptomatic and symptomatic left ventricular systolic dysfunction: a retrospective analysis of the SOLVD trials. *J Am Coll Cardiol* 1998; **32**: 695–703.

Krahn AD, Klein GJ, Kerr CR *et al*. How useful is thyroid function testing in patients with recent-onset atrial fibrillation? *Arch Intern Med* 1996; **156**: 2221–4.

Krahn AD, Manfreda J, Tate RB *et al*. The natural history of atrial fibrillation: Incidence, risk factors, and prognosis in the Manitoba Follow-up Study. *Am J Med* 1995; **98**: 476.

Lip GYH, Golding DJ, Nazir M *et al*. A survey of atrial fibrillation in general practice: the west Birmingham Atrial Fibrillation Project. *Br J Gen Pract* 1997; **47**: 285–9.

Lip GYH, Tean KN, Dunn FG. Treatment of atrial fibrillation in a district general hospital. *Br Heart J* 1994; **71**: 92–5.

Van den Berg MP, Tuinenburg AE, Crijns HJ *et al*. Heart failure and atrial fibrillation: current concepts and controversies. *Heart* 1997; **77**: 309–13.

Wheeldon NM, Tayler DI, Anagnostou E *et al*. Screening for atrial fibrillation in primary care. *Heart* 1998; **79**: 50–5.

Zarifis J, Beevers DG, Lip GYH. Acute admissions with atrial fibrillation in a British multiracial hospital population. *Br J Clin Pract* 1997; **51**: 91–6.

3. Pathophysiology and electrophysiology

Pathophysiology
Electrophysiology

Pathophysiological consequences of AF

- Usually relate to loss of effective atrial systolic function ('atrial kick') and atrioventricular synchrony.
- Both effectively reduce stroke volume and cardiac output, especially in the presence of structural heart disease.
- The loss of atrial systolic function results in two main sequelae:

  impaired haemodynamic function of the heart

  intra-atrial stasis and thrombogenesis, predisposing to stroke and thromboembolism.

Pathophysiology

Loss of atrial systolic function and a fast, irregular, ventricular response result in impairment of haemodynamic function. Thus, atrial fibrillation (AF) is a less efficient cardiac rhythm, and accounts for the symptoms of reduced exercise tolerance, such as fatigue, lethargy etc. This is partially compensated by a fast heart rate, which may lead to palpitations, chest pain, giddiness or syncope, shortness of breath and anxiety. In more severe cases, the haemodynamic effects can result in heart failure.

The loss of atrial systole by the change in rhythm from sinus rhythm to AF in patients with significant diastolic dysfunction, with stiff, non-compliant ventricles (for example, in left ventricular hypertrophy or hypertrophic cardiomyopathy), can result in heart failure.

While heart disease (eg mitral valve disease, hypertension) can lead to a dilated left atrium in AF, there is evidence that AF itself can result in progressive dilatation of the left atrium.

Prolonged fast AF can alter the myocardium electrophysiologically and ultrastructurally, resulting in dilatation and reduction of systolic function, commonly referred to as 'tachycardia-induced cardiomyopathy' or 'tachycardiomyopathy'. These can be associated with ultrastructural abnormalities visualized on electron microscopy. Thus, fast AF with poor heart rate control can result in progressive cardiac enlargement and worsening heart failure.

The presence of AF results in intra-atrial stasis, which increases the risk of thrombus formation, usually in the left atrial appendage. This stasis is typically visualized as the phenomenon of spontaneous echocontrast, which is characterized by swirling shadows in the left atrium, seen usually with transoesophageal echocardiography (TEE), and reduced left atrial appendage flow velocities. There are also abnormalities of haemostasis and coagulation in AF, resulting in a prothrombotic or hypercoagulable state, as well as evidence of atrial endocardial damage, which all contribute to abnormalities of Virchow's triad and increased thrombogenesis in AF (Figure 3.1).

Abnormal flow – dilated LA, atrial stasis, associated heart failure, hypertension, etc.

Abnormal blood constituents
– clotting factors
– platelets

Abnormal vessel wall
– atrial endocardial damage/dysfunction
– endothelial damage dysfunction

Figure 3.1
Atrial fibrillation and Virchow's triad.

Pathophysiological classifications

AF may be classified according to its aetiology and underlying disease, its electrophysiological features or its temporal pattern. For example, AF is commonly classified (aetiologically) into valvular or non-valvular varieties. This was particularly useful when rheumatic heart disease was common and it accounted for many cases of AF in younger people. Other aetiologies are used to categorize AF: ischaemic, alcoholic and thyrotoxic are useful as they focus attention on the need to deal with underlying disease rather than the AF alone.

Some patients with paroxysmal AF have autonomic influences on paroxysms, and have been described as having 'vagotonic' or 'adrenergic' AF. Many patients present with an intermediate or mixed pattern. Perhaps as much as one-quarter of paroxysmal AF is vagotonic, and one-fifth is the adrenergic form.

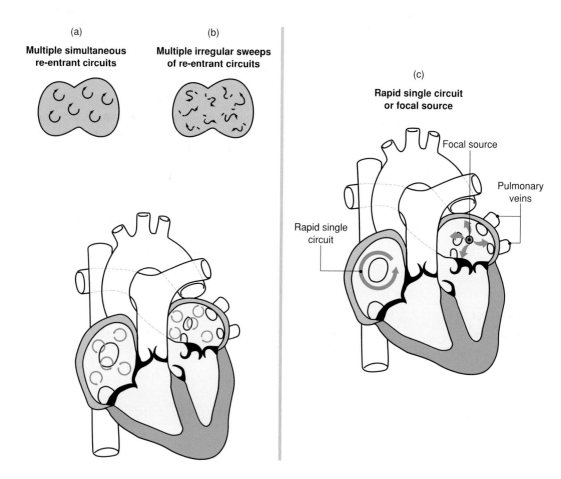

Figure 3.2
Electrophysiology of atrial fibrillation. (a) Moe's model (1962), (b) Allesie's model (1970s), and (c) 'focal AF'.

Vagotonic AF	Adrenergic AF
• Typically affects younger patients with no underlying structural heart disease	• Typically affects older patients; often associated with mild to moderate structural heart disease
• Post-prandial or evening or nocturnal paroxysms	• Attacks occur during or after exercise, with alcohol, etc
• Tends not to progress to established forms of AF	• May become established
• Usually occurs with a slow ventricular rate	• Usually occurs with a fast ventricular rate
• Beta-blockers and digoxin less useful, whereas Class Ic (eg flecainide) and III (eg amiodarone) are drugs of choice	• Beta-blockers and digoxin useful

Electrophysiology

The electrophysiological mechanism(s) of AF are thought to involve several coexisting re-entrant wavefronts usually in abnormal atrial tissue, whether or not enlarged (secondary to mitral valve disease, hypertension, etc), fibrosed (resulting in slowing of intra-atrial conduction) or with altered autonomic tone, especially increased sympathetic activity (Figure 3.2). In addition, heterogeneity of atrial refractoriness and slow conduction times (allowing time for the myocardium to regain excitability between each wavefront) help perpetuate the process, leading to AF being sustained in the long term.

Moe's model in 1962 proposed multiple coexisting re-entrant wavefronts of activation in the atria. More recently, Allesie's model (1970s) suggested that AF was due to multiple wavelets continuously sweeping around the atria in irregular shifting patterns, repeatedly encountering excitable myocardium. Further appreciation of the electrophysiological mechanisms have identified 'focal AF' where paroxysmal AF originates from an abnormal focus in the pulmonary veins, which can result in cure by the ablation of this area. Stabilization of the atria electrophysiologically by atrial pacing during the sick sinus syndrome can prevent paroxysms of AF.

The atria may also be altered electrophysiologically by prolonged episodes of AF, resulting in even longer paroxysms and greater difficulty in reversion back to sinus rhythm. This is the concept of 'AF begets AF' and was elegantly shown by Allesie's group in a goat model of pacing-induced AF.

Pathophysiology and electrophysiology of AF		
Haemodynamic	*Thrombogenic*	*Electro-mechanical*
Fast and irregular rhythm	Stasis	'AF begets AF' –
Tachycardia-induced cardiomyopathy	Endocardial/endothelial remodelling	electrophysical abnormalities
Atrial dilatation	Abnormal haemostasis	
Structural heart disease	Platelets	

Further reading

Allessie MA, Konings K, Kirchhof CJHJ, Wijffels M. Electrophysiologic mechanisms of perpetuation of atrial fibrillation. *Am J Cardiol* 1996; **77**:10A.

Gallagher MM, Obel OA, Camm JA. Tachycardia-induced atrial myopathy: an important mechanism in the pathophysiology of atrial fibrillation? *J Cardiovasc Electrophysiol* 1997; **8**: 1065–74.

Goette A, Honeycutt C, Langberg JJ. Electrical remodeling in atrial fibrillation. *Circulation* 1996; **94**: 2968.

Haissaguerre M, Jais P, Shah DC *et al.* Spontaneous initiation of atrial fibrillation by ectopic beats originating in the pulmonary veins. *N Engl J Med* 1998; **339**: 659–66.

Jais P, Haissaguerre M, Shah DC *et al.* A focal source of atrial fibrillation treated by discrete radiofrequency ablation. *Circulation* 1997; **95**: 572.

Lip GYH. Does atrial fibrillation confer a hypercoagulable state? *Lancet* 1995; **346**: 1313–4.

Lip GYH. Hypercoagulability and haemodynamic abnormalities in atrial fibrillation. *Heart* 1997; **77**: 395-6.

Li Saw Hee FL, Blann AD, Goldsmith I, Lip GYH. Indices of hypercoagulability measured in peripheral blood reflect levels in intracardiac blood in patients with atrial fibrillation secondary to mitral stenosis. *Am J Cardiol* 1999; **83**: 1206–9.

Moe GK. On the multiple wavelet hypothesis of atrial fibrillation. *Arch Int Pharmacodyn Ther* 1962; **140**: 183.

Tieleman RG, De Langen CDJ, Van Gelder IC *et al.* Verapamil reduces tachycardia-induced electrical remodeling of the atria. *Circulation* 1997; **95**: 1945.

Wijffels MCEF, Kirchhof CJHJ, Dorland R *et al.* Atrial fibrillation begets atrial fibrillation. A study in awake chronically instrumented goats. *Circulation* 1995; **92**: 1954.

4. Clinical features

Symptoms
Clinical examination
Overview

- AF can be symptomatic or asymptomatic.
- Both symptomatic and asymptomatic episodes of AF can occur in the same patient.
- The clinical features of AF relate to haemodynamic and thromboembolic complications, as well as the morbidity associated with therapy (drugs, devices, and so on).

A patient initially presenting with atrial fibrillation may do so acutely or as a more chronic rhythm disorder, which can be symptomatic or asymptomatic. Most patients (90%) in AF who are referred to outpatients have symptoms. Asymptomatic AF is usually discovered incidentally during pulse-taking, cardiac auscultation or 12-lead ECG recording or 24-hour Holter recording undertaken for unrelated reasons. In one comparison of patients with paroxysmal supraventricular tachycardia (PSVT) and

The clinical history in a new presentation with AF should include the following:
- Date of the first episode
- Information about acute precipitating factors or chronic conditions linked to AF
- How symptoms are relieved
- Typical duration of and interval between episodes
- Duration of the current or last episode
- Previous drug treatment

patients with paroxysmal AF, most episodes of PSVT tended to be symptomatic, while only one in 12 paroxysms of AF were symptomatic.

Symptoms

No studies have been found regarding sensitivity or specificity of symptoms in detecting AF. However, a French survey of 756 patients with electrocardiographically documented AF found that 89.6% had symptoms of some description, principally palpitations (54.1%) and dyspnoea (44.4%). The prevalence of asymptomatic AF in the community is unknown.

Symptoms associated with AF can vary depending on several factors, including the ventricular rate, cardiac function, concomitant co-morbid medical problems and individual patient perception. Some patients with AF have few symptoms, but many will present with haemodynamic-related symptoms (such as tiredness, fatigue, reduced exercise tolerance and those related to heart failure) and more serious complications, such as heart failure or thromboembolism. If the patient complains of angina, it should be established whether or not the angina occurs only during attacks of AF due to an uncontrolled ventricular rate or whether or not angina occurs independently of the arrhythmia. Shortness of breath may be due to pulmonary oedema, and giddiness or syncope due to associated hypotension.

Palpitations in patients with AF may be due to awareness of a fast heart rate or slow irregular rate. The duration of AF may be unknown in many patients, and whether or not AF was the cause or effect of, eg heart failure, may be uncertain.

Clinical examination

On physical examination, AF is typically associated with an irregularly irregular pulse. A careful history and clinical examination will often reveal underlying medical problems associated with AF, such as hypertension, ischaemic heart disease, valvular heart disease and cardiomyopathy. It should be remembered that common non-cardiac factors such as excessive alcohol, thyroid disease, chest disease and any infection or pyrexial illness can precipitate AF. Very often the patient presents because of medical problems associated with AF, such as heart failure or stroke, and will have these features on clinical examination. Very rarely, right-sided thrombi may lead to pulmonary thromboembolism.

Signs of atrial fibrillation

The Newcastle survey assessed screening methods for the presence of AF in an age-stratified sample of 1,235 subjects aged >65 years using a screening limb lead ECG, and reported that the sensitivity of pulse palpation was 93–100% and specificity 71–86%, being lower in more elderly groups. There was little benefit found from adding a prescription of digoxin as a screening criterion.

Standard teaching is that the pulse in AF is irregularly irregular in rate and volume. Rawles et al studied the rhythm and character of pulse in 74 patients, 36 of whom were taking digoxin: 30% of AF patients were found to have regularity of rhythm and 59% of cases had regularity of pulse volume (that is, the sequence of consecutive pulse volumes was significantly non-random). The use of digoxin did not effect regularity or otherwise of pulse.

Escudero et al studied 32 patients with AF using ECG (for relative risk [RR] interval) and carotid pulse and found that the irregularity of pulse was maintained despite varying ventricular rates whereas the inequality between beats was reduced at slower ventricular rates. Sneed et al studied the ability of nurses to count accurately the pulse of patients with AF over 15, 30 and 60 seconds at both apical and radial pulses, which was compared to both simultaneous electrocardiographic (ECG) and plethysmographic (pleth) recordings as reference standards. They found that the apical method was significantly more accurate than the radial method, regardless of whether or not the ECG or pleth standard was used (ECG, $p<0.0001$; pleth, $p=0.036$); furthermore, the 60-second counting interval was significantly more accurate, regardless of the standard (ECG, $p=0.006$; pleth, $p=0.02$).

Overview

A careful clinical history from a patient with AF should lay emphasis on certain clinical features, such as whether or not symptoms are intermittent or sustained, when or how did they first start, and any associated complications, such as heart failure, stroke or thromboembolism. Alcohol is another common precipitant of acute-onset AF, especially in younger patients, which is commonly overlooked but could be elicited from a careful history. Occult or manifest thyrotoxicosis should be considered, especially in the elderly patient with AF, where the signs of thyrotoxicosis may be less apparent. Heart failure is associated with AF in approximately one-third of patients, and since each can lead to the other, and both are commonly related to underlying heart disease, it could be difficult to ascertain the precise aetiological factor.

Further reading

Escudero EM, Iveli CA, Moreyra AE et al. The pulse in patients with atrial fibrillation: its irregularity and inequality. Euro J Cardio 1976; **4**: 31–8.

Levy S, Maarek M, Coumel P et al. Characterization of different subsets of atrial fibrillation in general practice in France: the ALFA study. The College of French Cardiologists. Circulation 1999; **99**: 3028–35.

Lip GYH, Tean KN, Dunn FG. Treatment of atrial fibrillation in a district general hospital. Br Heart J 1994; **71**: 92–5.

Page RL, Wilkinson WE, Clair WK et al. Asymptomatic arrhythmias in patients with symptomatic paroxysmal atrial fibrillation and paroxysmal supraventricular tachycardia. Circulation 1994; **89**: 224–7.

Rawles JM. What is meant by a 'controlled' ventricular rate in atrial fibrillation? Br Heart J 1990; **63**: 157–61.

Sneed NV, Hollerbach AD. Accuracy of heart rate assessment in atrial fibrillation. Heart Lung 1992; **21**: 427–33.

Sudlow M, Rodgers H, Kenny RA, Thomson R. Identification of patients with atrial fibrillation in general practice: a study of screening methods. BMJ 1998; **317**: 327–8.

5. Investigations

Basic investigations
Documenting the arrhythmia
Echocardiography
Other investigations

Investigations in a patient with AF

- When assessing a patient with possible AF, it is important to document the arrhythmia, and confirm whether or not the patient actually has AF.

- As AF commonly occurs in association with other cardiac and non-cardiac disease, investigations are necessary to identify and correct potentially treatable causes.

Basic investigations

- A full blood count is useful, especially when antithrombotic therapy is considered.

- Serum urea and electrolytes are relevant before considering some drug therapies (for example, a reduced dose of digoxin in renal impairment or ACE inhibitors for associated heart failure).

- Thyroid function tests should be measured in all patients with atrial fibrillation (AF) even if there are no symptoms suggestive of thyrotoxicosis, as subclinical thyroid disease is often present in the elderly and AF may be its first presentation.

- A chest X-ray may occasionally be useful in patients with AF. For example, the chest X-ray can give information on heart size and the presence of pulmonary oedema,

intrathoracic pathology or even pericardial disease. In the young patient with AF, the chest X-ray may provide a clue to congenital heart disease, such as atrial septal defect.

Documenting the arrhythmia

It is inadvisable to start drugs without any documentation of the arrhythmia. A 12-lead 'standard' ECG may suffice to document the arrhythmia (Figures 5.1, 5.2). The ECG in AF typically shows atrial activity as irregular baseline undulations of varying amplitude and morphology, which are referred to as 'f' (fibrillation) waves and could be as fast as 600/min. The ventricular complexes are irregularly irregular – the rate is rarely as fast as the atrial rate since the atrioventricular node is unable to conduct impulses at this fast rate unless impulses are conducted through accessory pathways. In long-standing AF, the ECG baseline may appear smooth without any P wave.

Rapid AF with a rapid ventricular response may be mistaken for other supraventricular arrhythmias (for example, atrial flutter or supraventricular tachycardias) or if a bundle branch block is present, ventricular tachycardia. Subtle variations in the relative risk (RR) interval are the important clues. The ECG may also provide a clue to the aetiology or electrophysiological features that may have caused the AF. For example, the presence of prior myocardial infarction, left ventricular hypertrophy or pre-excitation syndromes (such as the delta wave in Wolff-Parkinson-White syndrome) may be seen on the 12-lead ECG.

If symptoms are intermittent and suggest paroxysmal AF, a 24-hour ambulatory ECG should provide the diagnosis if they occur on a daily basis. However, if symptoms occur less frequently, a patient-activated event recorder ('Cardiomemo', Figures 5.3 and 5.4) would be more effective. Certainly, only a minority of paroxysms of AF are symptomatic

(a)

(b)

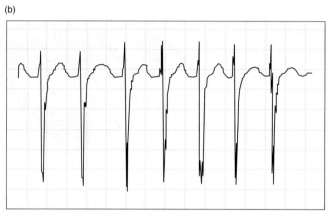

Figure 5.1
ECGs showing (a) controlled AF and (b) fast AF.

(a)

(b)

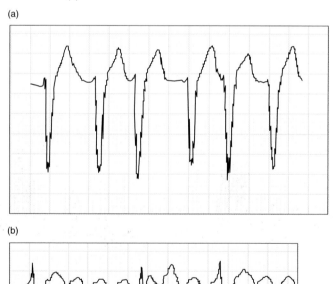

Figure 5.2
ECGs showing (a) AF with bundle branch block and (b) atrial flutter.

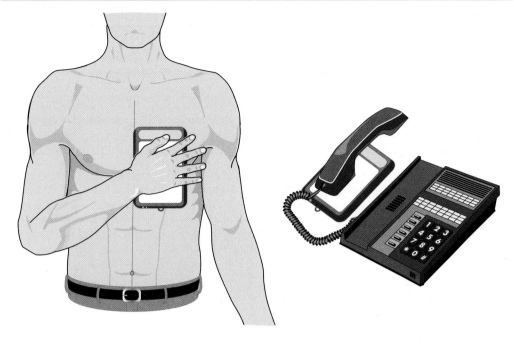

Recording an ECG   ECG transmission

Figure 5.3
Cardiomemo.

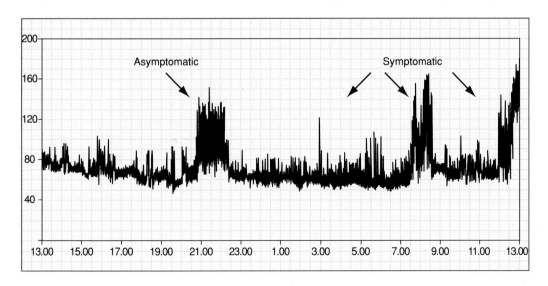

Figure 5.4
Paroxysmal AF 24-hour heart rate profile.

but the optimal management of asymptomatic paroxysms of AF is uncertain (see chapter 8).

Echocardiography

Most cardiologists would request a transthoracic echocardiogram for the initial evaluation of most patients with AF. Although transthoracic echocardiography is adequate for assessing chamber size, detection of atrial thrombi or the assessment of left atrial appendage anatomy and/or function requires transoesophageal echocardiography (TOE), especially if a prosthetic mitral valve is present or in cases where transthoracic imaging is inadequate.

Transthoracic echocardiographic features associated with a high risk of stroke and thromboembolism in the Stroke Prevention in AF (SPAF)-I study included left atrial dilatation (corrected for body surface area) and poor left ventricular function. Nevertheless, in their recent overview of echocardiographic data from 1066 patients from three clinical trials, the AF investigators reported that isolated left atrial enlargement *per se* was not an independent risk factor for stroke on multivariate analysis, although moderate to severe left ventricular systolic dysfunction on two-dimensional echocardiography did appear to be a predictor. In the SPAF-III transoesophageal echocardiography substudy, features associated with a high risk of stroke included the presence of spontaneous echo contrast, thrombus in left atrial appendage and complex aortic plaques.

Echocardiography therefore complements risk stratification for stroke and thromboembolic risk on clinical grounds, and should be useful in a small group of patients who have a low risk of stroke according to clinical risk factors. This is confirmed by the Newcastle survey data where echocardiography was useful in deciding the need for warfarin in the small proportion of subjects with AF who did not have clinical risk factors.

Many subjects with AF in whom transthoracic echocardiography detected 'high risk' features often have one or more clinical risk factors for thromboembolism, and thus, echocardiography usually did not alter antithrombotic therapy management.

Echocardiography in AF

- To establish the presence of structural heart disease (including valvular abnormalities, congenital anomalies, chamber dimensions, pericardial thickening or effusions).
- To assess ventricular function.
- To decide on the suitability for cardioversion.
- To aid thromboembolic risk stratification.
- Transoesophageal echocardiography-guided cardioversion is one option for patients with AF who need cardioversion but wish to minimize anticoagulation duration and complications.

Other investigations

Exercise testing may occasionally be needed in order to clarify the severity of underlying cardiac ischaemia, although caution in interpretation of the ST segments may be needed in patients taking digoxin or if left ventricular hypertrophy is present.

Invasive electrophysiological studies usually have a limited role in the routine evaluation of most patients with AF. Electrophysiological studies in patients with AF should be reserved for those patients with associated electrophysiological abnormalities (including pre-excitation, sinus node dysfunction, etc) who could potentially benefit from the investigation and a curative electrophysiological procedure.

Table 5.1

Minimum and additional clinical evaluations in patients with AF: ACC/AHA/ESC guidelines for the management of patients with atrial fibrillation

Minimum evaluation

1. History and physical examination, to define:
- The presence and nature of symptoms associated with AF
- The clinical type of AF (first episode, paroxysmal, persistent or permanent)
- The onset of the first symptomatic attack or date of discovery of AF
- The frequency, duration, precipitating factors and modes of termination of AF
- The response to any pharmacological agents that have been administered
- The presence of any underlying heart disease or other reversible conditions (eg hyperthyroidism or alcohol consumption)

2. Electrocardiogram, to identify:
- Rhythm (verify AF)
- LV hypertrophy
- P-wave duration and morphology or fibrillatory waves
- Pre-excitation
- Bundle-branch block
- Prior MI
- Other atrial arrhythmias
- To measure and follow the RR, QRS and QT intervals in conjunction with antiarrhythmic drug therapy

3. Chest radiograph, to evaluate:
- The lung parenchyma, when clinical findings suggest an abnormality
- The pulmonary vasculature, when clinical findings suggest an abnormality

4. Echocardiogram, to identify:
- Valvular disease
- Left and right atrial size
- LV size and function
- Peak RV pressure (pulmonary hypertension)
- LV hypertrophy
- LA thrombus (low sensitivity)
- Pericardial disease

5. Blood tests of thyroid function
- For a first episode of AF, when the ventricular rate is difficult to control, or when AF recurs unexpectedly after cardioversion

Additional testing

One or several tests may be necessary

1. Exercise testing
- If the adequacy of rate control is in question (permanent AF)
- To reproduce exercise-induced AF
- To exclude ischaemia before treatment of selected patients with a type IC antiarrhthymic drug

2. Holter monitoring or event recording
- If diagnosis of the type of arrhythmia is in question
- As a means of evaluating rate control

3. Transoesophageal echocardiography
- To identify LA thrombus (in the LA appendage)
- To identify a predisposing arrhythmia such as atrial flutter or paroxysmal supraventricular tachycardia
- Seeking sites for curative ablation or AV conduction block/modification

AF=atrial fibrillation; LV=left ventricular; MI=myocardial infarction; RV=right ventricular; LA=left atrial; AV=atrioventricular. Type IC refers to the Vaughan–Williams classification of antiarrhythmic drugs.

Further reading

Atrial Fibrillation Investigators. Echocardiographic predictors of stroke in patients with atrial fibrillation: A prospective study of 1,066 patients from three clinical trials. *Arch Intern Med* 1998; **158**: 1316–20.

Black IW, Hopkins AP, Lee LC *et al*. Left atrial spontaneous echo contrast: A clinical and echocardiographic analysis. *J Am Coll Cardiol* 1991; **18**: 398.

Dittrich HC, Erickson JS, Schneiderman T *et al*. Echocardiographic and clinical predictors for outcome of elective cardioversion of atrial fibrillation. *Am J Cardiol* 1989; **63**: 193.

Forfar JC. Atrial fibrillation and the pituitary-thyroid axis: a re-evaluation. *Heart* 1997; **77**(1): 3–4.

Fuster V, Ryden LE, Asinger RW *et al*. ACC/AHA/ESC guidelines for the management of patients with atrial fibrillation: executive summary. A Report of the American College of Cardiology/ American Heart Association Task Force on Practice Guidelines and the European Society of Cardiology Committee for Practice Guidelines and Policy Conferences (Committee to Develop Guidelines for the Management of Patients With Atrial Fibrillation): developed in Collaboration with the North American Society of Pacing and Electrophysiology. *J Am Coll Cardiol* 2001; **38**(4): 1231–66.

Klein AL, Grimm RA, Black IW *et al*. Cardioversion guided by transesophageal echocardiography: the ACUTE Pilot Study. A randomized, controlled trial. Assessment of cardioversion using transesophageal echocardiography. *Ann Intern Med* 1997; **126**: 200–9.

Lip GYH. How would I manage a 60-year old woman presenting with atrial fibrillation? *Proc R Coll Physicians Edinb* 1999; **29**: 301–6.

Stoddard ME, Dawkins PR, Prince CR, Ammash NM. Left atrial appendage thrombus is not uncommon in patients with acute atrial fibrillation and a recent embolic event: a transesophageal echocardiographic study. *J Am Coll Cardiol* 1995; **25**: 452–9.

Stroke Prevention in Atrial Fibrillation Committee on Echocardiography. Transesophageal echocardiographic correlates of thromboembolism in high-risk patients with atrial fibrillation. *Ann Intern Med* 1998; **128**: 639–47.

Stroke Prevention in Atrial Fibrillation Investigators. Predictors of thromboembolism in atrial fibrillation: II. Echocardiographic features of patients at risk. *Ann Intern Med* 1992; **116**: 6–12.

Sudlow M, Thomson R, Thwaites B *et al*. Prevalence of atrial fibrillation and eligibility for anticoagulants in the community. *Lancet* 1998; **325**: 1167–71.

6. Non-drug management

Pacemaker therapy
Electrophysiological techniques
Atrial implantable defibrillator
(atrioverter)
Surgery

Non-pharmacological measures for AF
- General measures – avoid precipitants, minimize alcohol intake, treat heart failure, etc.
- Electrophysiological techniques – atrioventricular node modification, atrioventricular node ablation ± pacemaker, 'catheter maze', focal AF ablation, atrial defibrillator (atrioverter), internal cardioversion, etc.
- Pacemaker – atrial pacing for sick sinus syndrome, biatrial pacing, etc.
- Surgery – maze and corridor procedures.

(See text for details and Table 6.2 for summary)

Particular advances in the non-drug management of atrial fibrillation (AF) have been directed at patients who have been poorly responsive to medical therapy. Developments in electrophysiology and surgery have allowed the possibility of a 'cure' for AF, in some instances, such as 'focal AF', where AF originates from pulmonary vein foci. However, as many interventions may be irreversible, such as atrioventricular node ablation, the decision should be made in consultation with a specialist cardiologist, and fully discussed with the patient. Strategies for control of heart rate in AF patients are compared in Table 6.1.

Pacemaker therapy

There have been great advances in pacemaker technology and sophistication with the development of new pacing algorithms, pacing modes (including mode-switching) etc. At the most basic level, a pacemaker system consists of lead electrodes implanted into the right atrium and/or right ventricle, and a pacemaker generator, which is implanted subcutaneously, usually over the pectoral region. Most generators are getting smaller in size, and have a lifetime of nearly a decade. Pacemaker clinics allow follow-up and computer interrogation of recent arrhythmic events and programming.

Table 6.1
Strategies for heart rate control in AF

	Control of resting heart rate	Control of exercise heart rate	Thrombo-embolic risk still present?	Symptomatic benefit	Haemodynamic benefit
Digoxin monotherapy	Yes	No	Yes	+	+
Digoxin + beta-blocker or calcium antagonist	Yes	Yes	Yes	++	+
Radiofrequency ablation + pacemaker	Yes	Yes	Yes	++	++
Radiofrequency modification	Yes	Yes	Yes	+++	+++

Basic pacemaker nomenclature

1st letter – chamber paced (V = ventricle;
A = atrium; D = double)

2nd letter – chamber sensed (V = ventricle;
A = atrium; D = double; 0 = none)

3rd letter – response to sensed impulse
(I = inhibitory, T = triggered; D = double;
0 = none)

4th letter – if 'R' = rate-responsive

Described simplistically...

- VVIR: single chamber, right ventricle sensed and paced, rate-responsive

- AAIR: single chamber, right atrium sensed and paced, rate responsive

- DDDR: dual chamber, both right atrium and right ventricle, senses and paced, rate-responsive

---

Pacemakers are indicated in AF for symptomatic low heart rates where anti-bradycardia pacing (usually VVIR pacing mode) is considered. A pacemaker may also be needed for chromotropic incompetence during exercise, that is, an inadequate heart rate response to exercise, resulting in significant limitation of the patient's exercise capacity, which requires a rate-adaptive VVIR pacemaker, even in the absence of significant bradycardia at rest.

Atrioventricular nodal ablation or atrioventricular nodal modification (that is, slow/fast pathway modification) for control of ventricular rate in patients with chronic or paroxysmal AF may result in atrioventricular block, requiring permanent pacing, usually with VVIR pacing mode.

In the sick sinus syndrome, there is a significant decrease in the incidence of AF with atrial pacing, perhaps by stabilizing the atria electrically. In addition, atrial pacing prevents the development of AF that occurs during bradycardia by suppressing the development of atrial premature beats, which can initiate AF when they occur. In the best studies of atrial pacing for sick sinus syndrome, atrial pacing (AAI or DDD mode) conferred a significantly lower risk of AF, thromboembolism, heart

failure and mortality compared to ventricular pacing at eight years of follow-up, and in those with intact atrioventricular conduction at baseline, there was only a low incidence of progression to atrioventricular block. In patients who have evidence of atrioventricular nodal disease, a dual chamber pacemaker is often preferred. Nevertheless, the use of dual chamber pacemakers may result in tracking of atrial rates to the upper rate limit of the pacemaker, which can be overcome by the use of a pacemaker with mode switching capability.

Multisite atrial pacing may be useful in AF prevention, by increasing the coupling interval of the initiating premature beat in the abnormal substrate either by pre-exciting the re-entry zone or by pacing at one or more sites that are opposite to the activation of the premature beat. However, more data in larger numbers of patients are clearly needed.

Pacemakers in AF – indications

- Symptomatic bradycardia which is related to atrioventricular block or the use of antiarrhythmic drugs

- Symptomatic chromotropic incompetence during exercise

- Acquired atrioventricular block from atrioventricular nodal ablation or from an attempt at atrioventricular nodal modification

- Sick sinus syndrome

Electrophysiological techniques

Atrioventricular node modification and 'ablate and pace'

In drug-resistant, poorly tolerated AF, atrioventricular (AV) junction modification to slow conduction through the AV node, or alternatively, catheter ablation with VVIR pacemaker implantation ('ablate and pace') is an option. For paroxysmal AF, DDDR mode-switching pacemaker is more appropriate.

'Ablate and pace' is highly effective in controlling the symptoms of AF, improving general wellbeing and quality of life, and increasing exercise capacity. However there is a risk of progression to permanent AF (thus, necessitating continuation of anticoagulation) and some series have even reported an increased risk of sudden death. A recent meta-analysis by Wood *et al* of 21 studies (1181 patients) reported that 'ablate and pace' was associated with improved outcomes in terms of symptoms, quality of life, cardiac function and healthcare use. However, only two of the studies were randomized trials and the comparison in the meta-analysis was to clinical outcomes before the therapy rather than to a control group.

Catheter maze

Radiofrequency ablation is used to create linear non-conductive barriers to prevent intra-atrial re-entry, commonly referred to as a 'catheter maze' procedure. While results are encouraging, the procedure is very lengthy and the radiation exposure is substantial.

Focal atrial fibrillation ablation

Some young patients with no detectable heart disease and AF due to a rapidly firing atrial foci located near the orifice of the pulmonary veins into the left atrium or in the left pulmonary veins have been treated by radiofrequency ablation of the atrial foci resulting in a 'cure' for these patients. There is a risk of pulmonary vein stenosis, and consequent pulmonary hypertension. This is an exciting new area and data from the largest centres are very encouraging.

Atrial implantable defibrillator (atrioverter)

Using technology similar to that used for suppression of ventricular tachyarrhythmias, the standalone atrioverter delivers low energy shocks (less than six joules) designed to re-establish sinus rhythm with a minimum risk of ventricular arrhythmias. This new therapy is currently under evaluation and the initial results are encouraging.

In an uncontrolled study, Wellens *et al* found that 96% of 227 spontaneous episodes of AF in 41 patients were successfully converted. The major problems with the atrioverter are chest pain after the device 'fires' (with shocks >1 joule) and the potential risk of inducing ventricular tachycardia or fibrillation. Nevertheless, the use of this device may provide significant symptom relief and improved quality of life in patients with paroxysmal AF who may have been very symptomatic as a result of their arrhythmia or may have experienced many side-effects with drug therapy.

Internal cardioversion

In patients resistant to external trans-thoracic cardioversion or pharmacological cardioversion, internal electrical cardioversion is a relatively new technique that has been showing fairly promising results. Electrodes are placed in, for example, the coronary sinus and right ventricle and a synchronized electrical shock is applied, with >90% success rates in previously resistant cases.

Surgery

Surgery is limited to a selected group of patients with AF who are often resistant to conventional treatment. As chronic AF often occurs in the setting of mitral and aortic valve disease, some patients may benefit from additional surgery for the cure of AF performed in combination with valve replacement surgery.

The goals of surgery for AF
- The abolition of AF
- Restoration of sinus rhythm
- The re-establishment or maintenance of atrioventricular synchrony (including restoration of atrial transport)
- The reduction or elimination of the risk of stroke and thromboembolism by reducing intra-atrial blood stasis

---

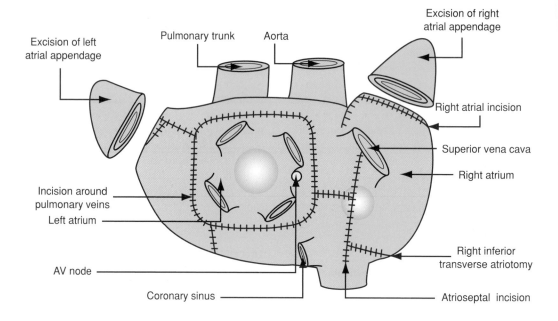

Figure 6.1
Maze procedure, with the heart viewed from behind.

Two surgical procedures, the modified Cox 'maze' procedure and the left atrial isolation or 'corridor' procedure have generally been used.

In the 'maze' operation (Figure 6.1), several small incisions are made in the atria, excising both atrial appendices and isolating the pulmonary veins, to obtain compartments that are small enough and unable to sustain AF, thus resulting in interruption of the potential re-entrant pathways required for AF. The procedure cures AF, restores atrioventricular synchrony, and preserves atrial transport function in 98% of patients, with a 2% mortality and only 9% of patients requiring subsequent antiarrhythmic medications, and was effective in patients undergoing mitral valve surgery. Postoperative atrial pacemakers were needed in 40% of cases, mostly for a preoperative sick sinus syndrome but occasionally for iatrogenic sinus node injury.

The 'corridor' operation isolates the sinus node

area, a strip of atrial tissue and the atrioventricular node from the remaining atrium, thereby allowing sinus rhythm to be sustained. Sinus node function and physiological rate control of heart rate is restored but atrial contraction or atrioventricular synchrony is not. Hence, the risk of thromboembolism remains with a requirement for anticoagulation. Most patients would maintain sinus rhythm and achieve rate control at follow-up, but some patients may require a pacemaker due to postoperative sinus node dysfunction.

Further reading

Andersen HR, Nielsen JC, Thomsen PE *et al*. Atrioventricular conduction during long-term follow-up of patients with sick sinus syndrome. *Circulation* 1998; **98**(13): 1315–21.

Andersen HR, Nielsen JC, Thomsen PEB *et al*. Long-term follow-up of patients from a randomised trial of atrial versus ventricular pacing for sick sinus syndrome. *Lancet* 1997; **350**: 1210.

Table 6.2

Non-pharmacological treatments for paroxysmal atrial fibrillation

Treatment modality	Advantage	Disadvantage
Atrial pacing algorithms	Preventative	Unproven
Multisite atrial pacing	Preventative	Unproven Complicated
Ablation of focal atrial Tachycardia (AT)/atrial fibrillation (AF) stenosis	Curative	Not known how often AT causes AF Risk of pulmonary vein obstruction
Surgical 'maze' procedure	Curative	Major surgery Postoperative sick sinus syndrome
Radiofrequency ablation 'maze'	Curative	Long difficult procedure Systemic thromboembolism
AV nodal ablation with mode switching dual chamber pacemaker	Effective	Does not maintain atrial function Risk of thromboembolism
Implantable atrial defibrillator	Effective	May not prevent AF episodes Pain/discomfort during defibrillation

Adapted from Waktare JEP, Camm AJ. *Proc R Coll Physicians Edinb* 1999; **29**(Suppl 6): 5–12.

Brignole M, Gianfranchi L, Menozzi C *et al.* Assessment of atrioventricular junction ablation and DDDR mode-switching pacemaker versus pharmacological treatment in patients with severely symptomatic paroxysmal atrial fibrillation: a randomized controlled study. *Circulation* 1997 Oct 21; **96**(8): 2617–24.

Cox JL, Boineau JP, Schuessler RB *et al.* A review of surgery for atrial fibrillation. *J Cardiovasc Electrophysiol* 1991; **2**: 541.

Darpo B, Walfridsson H, Aunes M *et al.* Incidence of sudden death after radiofrequency ablation of the atrioventricular junction for atrial fibrillation. *Am J Cardiol* 1997 Nov 1; **80**(9): 1174–7.

Jais P, Haissaguerre M, Shah DC *et al.* A focal source of atrial fibrillation treated by discrete radiofrequency ablation. *Circulation* 1997 Feb 4; **95**(3): 572–6.

Saksena S, Prakash A, Hill M *et al.* Prevention of recurrent atrial fibrillation with chronic dual-site right atrial pacing. *J Am Coll Cardiol* 1996; **28**: 687.

Wellens HJ, Lau CP, Luderitz B *et al.* Atrioverter: an implantable device for the treatment of atrial fibrillation. *Circulation* 1998 Oct 20; **98**(16): 1651–6.

Wood MA *et al.* Clinical outcomes after ablation and pacing therapy for AF: a meta-analysis. *Circulation* 2000; **101**: 1138–44.

7. Drug management

Cardiac glycosides
Comparisons of antiarrhythmic agents
Class I antiarrhythmic agents
Class II antiarrhythmic agents
Class III antiarrhythmic agents
Class IV antiarrhythmic agents
Clonidine
Are antiarrhythmics all equal in terms of prognosis in AF patients?
Drugs for AF and heart failure

Pharmacological treatments can be used to restore and to maintain sinus rhythm and to control the ventricular rate in atrial fibrillation (AF). A wide range of drugs with different pharmacodynamic and pharmacokinetic properties can be used for the management of AF. Sometimes a combination of different groups of drugs may be needed for optimal management. These drugs do not 'cure' or abolish AF, but usually merely control or suppress it – this therapeutic goal needs to be made absolutely clear to the patient.

The most common used classification to describe the various drugs used is the Vaughan–Williams classification (Table 7.1), although a more mechanistic classification, called the 'Sicilian Gambit' classification, has been proposed.

The choice of drug used is dependent upon many factors, and certain general principles can be applied (Table 7.2).

Table 7.1
Vaughan–Williams classification

	Action	Examples
Class Ia		
Na+ channel blockers	Prolongs the action potential	Quinidine, procainamide, disopyramide
Class Ib		
Na+ channel blockers	Shortens the action potential	Lignocaine, mexiletine, phenytoin
Class Ic		
Na+ channel blockers	No significant effect on the action potential	Flecainide, encainide, propafenone, moracizine
Class II	Beta-adrenergic blockers	Propranolol, timolol, atenolol
Class III	Potassium channel blockers that prolong repolarization	Amiodarone, D-sotalol, L-sotalol, dofetilide, beryllium, ibutilide
Class IV	Slow calcium channel blockers	Verapamil, diltiazem, nifedipine

Note: some important antiarrhythmic drugs that are not included in the classification are digoxin and adenosine, which act predominantly by inhibiting the Na+/K+ pump and adenosine receptors, respectively.

Table 7.2
Antiarrhythmic drugs for AF: general principles

Management strategy	Class of drug
● Paroxysmal AF	Class Ia, Class Ic, Class II, Class III drugs
● Cardioversion of AF to sinus rhythm	Class Ia, Class Ic and Class III drugs
● Rate control	Class II, Class III, Class IV and digoxin
● Maintenance of sinus rhythm post cardioversion of AF	Class Ia, Class Ic, Class II, Class III drugs

Factors that determine the choice of the drug for AF

- Nature of AF (paroxysmal or sustained)
- Treatment strategy (cardioversion or rate control)
- Co-morbid conditions (obstructive airway disease etc)
- Ischaemic and/or structural heart disease
- The rapidity with which treatment is indicated
- Patient preference

A Cochrane systematic review of pharmacological interventions for AF is currently in preparation to address these issues. An evidence-based appraisal of drugs used for acute AF has recently been published in *Clinical Evidence*. However, drugs commonly used in AF (Table 7.3.) and the influence of co-morbid conditions are summarized on p. 35.

Table 7.3
Drugs commonly used in atrial fibrillation

	Route of administration	Loading dose (if required)	Maintenance dose
Class I			
Quinidine	Oral	Nil	200–400 mg 3–4 times daily
Flecainide	Oral	Nil	50 mg twice daily Maximum 150 mg twice daily
Flecainide	Intravenous	2 mg/kg over 10–30 min Maximum: 150 mg	1.5 µg/kg/h up to a maximum of 600 mg/day
Propafenone	Oral	Nil	150 mg three times/day increased gradually over days to maximum of 300 mg three times daily (if >70 kg)
Class II			
(eg) Metoprolol	Oral	Nil	25–100 mg x 2
	Intravenous	5–15 mg, at rate 1–2 mg/min	
Class III			
Sotalol	Oral*	Nil	40 mg twice daily increased gradually over days to maximum of 160 mg twice daily
Amiodarone	Oral	200 mg three times daily for one week; 200 mg twice daily for next week	200 mg/day
	Intravenous	5 mg/kg over 20–120 min	Maximum 1.2 g/day (including loading dose)
Class IV			
Diltiazem	Oral*	60–180 mg three times daily (unless long-acting preparation)	
Verapamil	Oral	Nil	40–160 mg x 3
	Intravenous	5–10 mg IV	
Digoxin	Oral	1–1.5 mg/day in divided doses	62.5–500 µg/day
	Intravenous	0.5–1 mg maximum given in fractions over 10–20 min up to four hourly	Nil

*Intravenous formulation not available in the UK.

Cardiac glycosides

Cardiac glycosides were first used by William Withering over 200 years ago, where the purple foxglove (*Digitalis purpurea*, which contains digitoxin) for the treatment of the 'dropsy', which is now recognized as cardiac failure, although many of his patients also had AF. Commercially available digoxin is obtained from the white foxglove, *Digitalis lanata*. Pharmacokinetic differences exist between digoxin and digitoxin, but the former is the more popular drug (in the UK, at least). An overview of digoxin for AF is summarized in the box.

Digoxin for AF

- Probably the most common antiarrhythmic agent prescribed for AF.
- Useful for ventricular rate control at rest (but not during exercise); and in AF with associated heart failure.
- May make paroxysmal AF worse, by increasing paroxysms and not controlling rate during paroxysms.
- Ineffective for cardioversion or the long-term maintenance of sinus rhythm postcardioversion.
- Ineffective, and can even be dangerous, in AF associated with pre-excitation, eg Wolff–Parkinson–White syndrome.
- Care needed when used in the elderly and in those with renal impairment.

Mechanism of action

The cardiac glycosides exert prominent vagotonic actions, resulting in the inhibition of calcium currents in the atrioventricular node, increasing the atrioventricular nodal refractoriness. The latter controls the ventricular rate in patients with AF. Digitalis also inhibits the Na^+/K^+ pump, causing the accumulation of intracellular Na^+. This Na^+ is exchanged for Ca^+ thus increasing the intracellular Ca^+ levels, providing cardiac ionotropic effects.

Clinical pharmacology

Digoxin can be administered both orally and intravenously. However, in acute AF, there is little advantage of giving digoxin intravenously except when the patient is unable to take oral tablets (for example, postoperatively) or there is probable malabsorption. Due to slow distribution and long half-life (36 hours), digoxin has a slow onset of action whether or not given orally or intravenously. More than 80% of digoxin undergoes renal elimination unchanged. This drug has a narrow therapeutic range and factors that predispose to toxicity include renal impairment, old age, and concurrent administration of other medication such as amiodarone and quinidine, hypokalaemia, hypercalcaemia and hypothyroidism.

Extracardiac manifestations of digoxin toxicity can include nausea, vomiting, visual disturbances such as yellow vision (xanthopsia), visual hallucinations and general confusion. Digitoxicity could induce any kind of cardiac arrhythmias, ranging from varying degrees of atrioventricular block, inhibition of the sino-atrial node, ventricular extrasystoles to ventricular tachycardia or fibrillation. Of the different arrhythmias seen in digitoxicity, paroxysmal atrial tachycardia with block is a characteristic feature.

Clinical use in atrial fibrillation

Clinically, digoxin and other cardiac glycosides are useful in controlling the resting ventricular rate in AF but control of the ventricular response in exercise and conditions of high sympathetic drive, such as uncontrolled heart failure, thyrotoxicosis, chronic lung disease, stress and pyrexia, is poor. Digoxin also has limited value in patients with AF secondary to an accessory pathway (such as the Wolff–Parkinson–White syndrome) and may even accelerate the ventricular response. Digoxin is no better than placebo in cardioverting AF to sinus rhythm and may even exacerbate paroxysmal AF by increasing the number of paroxysms, which tend to occur at faster heart rates. However, one recent double blind, cross-over, placebo-controlled trial of digoxin in 43 patients with symptomatic paroxysmal AF reported that digoxin reduces the frequency of symptomatic AF episodes, although the effect was small, with a median time to two episodes being 13.5 days on placebo and 18.7 days on digoxin.

Digoxin-resistant AF

- Not taking tablets
- Accessory pathway present, eg Wolff–Parkinson–White syndrome
- Thyrotoxicosis
- Poor left ventricular function
- Respiratory disease (including cor pulmonale and lung cancer)
- Metabolic and electrolyte abnormalities, hypoxia

Digoxin toxicity

- Common in elderly
- Renal impairment
- Electrolyte abnormalities, eg diuretic use resulting in hypokalaemia
- Drug interactions, eg quinidine, amiodarone
- Role for therapeutic drug monitoring

Comparisons of antiarrhythmic agents

This is a rapidly expanding field and newer antiarrhythmic agents are regularly involved for the management of AF. In trials that have compared antiarrhythmic agents to controls, a

US Department of Health and Human Services systematic review reported that quinidine, flecainide, propafenone, amiodarone, and ibutilide/dofetilide were all effective in AF rhythm control; there were insufficient data on disopyramide, and sotalol was shown to be ineffective. In trials comparing different antiarrhythmic agents, the evidence was strongest for flecainide, ibutilide/dofetilide, and propafenone.

The review by McNamara et al identified 45 trials evaluating 17 different agents for rate control in AF and concluded that the calcium channel blockers dilitiazem and verapamil were more effective than placebo or digoxin in reducing heart rate at rest and during exercise. Beta-blockers also reduced heart rate during rest and exercise, but were associated with reduced exercise tolerance in a number of studies. The evidence on digoxin was inconclusive.

Another meta-analysis of trials by Zarembski et al that included amiodarone or flecainide in the treatment of chronic (ie more than two weeks' duration) AF. They found six trials of amiodarone (315 patients) and two of flecainide (163 patients), and indirect comparison suggested that amiodarone was more effective at maintaining sinus rhythm up to one year. Southworth et al performed a meta-analysis of 10 studies that involved quinidine and four that involved sotalol, and indirect comparisons suggested that quinidine and sotalol achieved comparable maintenance rates of sinus rhythm at six months. There was a trend for both agents to increase mortality as compared to control. Indeed, a meta-analysis of trials of quinidine for maintenance of sinus rhythm found that while quinidine is effective at maintaining sinus rhythm, it was associated with increased mortality.

Class I antiarrhythmic agents

Class I antiarrhythmics remain popular drugs for use in AF. However, many Class I agents have serious adverse side-effects, including pro-arrhythmic properties, associated with prolongation of the QT interval and polymorphic ventricular tachycardia (*torsades de pointes*). Many of these drugs need to be initiated under medical supervision.

Class Ia

Class Ia agents are popular drugs in the US, although in the UK they have been largely superseded by the Class Ic agents. The Class Ia agents have an inhibitory effect on the sinus node function and the cardiac conducting tissue, leading to heart block or sinus arrest, and thus they should be used cautiously in patients with evidence of these abnormalities. In addition to their Class I antiarrhythmic properties, these drugs often have ancillary effects. For example, quinidine has an alpha-adrenergic blocking action and a mild anticholinergic effect. Disopyramide also has significant dose-related anticholinergic activity, which can cause urinary retention, constipation, dry mouth, oesophageal reflux and precipitation of acute glaucoma. Great care must be employed in administering disopyramide to somebody with urinary outflow obstruction and glaucoma or even a family history of glaucoma.

The anticholinergic action of the Class Ia agents may facilitate conduction through the atrioventricular node and on occasion, treatment leads to 1:1 conduction through the atrioventricular node resulting in a very fast ventricular rate. This is more common with atrial flutter and in young subjects with intact atrioventricular conduction, and concomitant administration of drugs such as beta-blockers, calcium channel blockers or digoxin is recommended. The alpha-blocking action of quinidine can cause vasodilatation, which could result in hypotension especially if nitrates and any other vasodilators are co-administered.

Proarrhythmia

- This is defined as the development of new arrhythmia or the worsening of the existing arrhythmia, following the institution of antiarrhythmic therapy at doses or plasma concentrations *below* those considered being toxic.
- Proarrhythmia is best avoided by removing the precipitating factor.

(*See Table 7.4 for details*)

Table 7.4

Types of proarrhythmia during treatment with various antiarrhythmic drugs for atrial fibrillation according to the Vaughan–Williams classification

Ventricular proarrhythmia
- Torsade de pointes (VW class Ia and class III drugs)
- Sustained monomorphic ventricular tachycardia (usually VW class Ic drugs)
- Sustained polymorphic ventricular tachycardia/VF without long QT (VW class Ia, Ic and III drugs)

Atrial proarrhythmia
- Provocation of recurrence (probably VW class Ia, Ic and III drugs)
- Conversion of AF to flutter (usually VW class Ic drugs)
- Increase of defibrillation threshold (a potential problem with VW class Ic drugs)

Abnormalities of conduction or impulse formation
- Acceleration of ventricular rate during AF (VW class Ia and class Ic drugs)
- Accelerate conduction over accessory pathways (digoxin, intravenous verapamil or diltiazem)
- Sinus node dysfunction, atrioventricular block (almost all drugs)

VW=Vaughan–Williams classification; VF=ventricular fibrillation.

Adapted with permission from Fuster V *et al. J Am Coll Cardiol* 2001; **38**(4): 1231–66. Copyright 2001 by the American College of Cardiology and the American Heart Association, Inc.

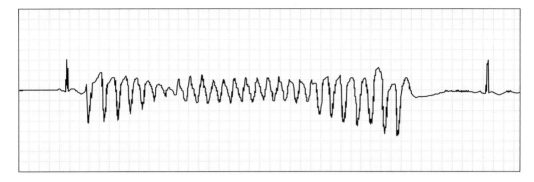

Figure 7.1
Torsade de pointes.

The major adverse effects associated with Class Ia agents also relate to proarrhythmia. For example, one meta-analysis of six randomized control trials comparing quinidine against placebo in maintaining sinus rhythm following cardioversion of AF demonstrated that quinidine was more effective than placebo (although only 50% in the quinidine group were still in sinus rhythm at one year) but was associated with higher mortality, which is likely to be related to proarrhythmia. The so-called 'quinidine syncope' is probably due to self-terminating *torsade de pointes* (Figure 7.1); this has been reported to occur each year in 1.5% of patients taking quinidine, and is unrelated to the plasma quinidine level or the duration of therapy, occurring when plasma concentrations are normal or below the therapeutic range.

Non-cardiac adverse effects of the Class Ia agents can include diarrhoea, nausea, vomiting and abdominal pain with quinidine. 'Cinchonism' is the term used to describe the cluster of neurological side-effects associated with quinidine, such as tinnitus, deafness, delirium, confusion. Procainamide is partly metabolized by acetylation in the liver and almost all patients on procainamide develop antinuclear antibodies; however in slow acetylators, 15–20% develop a lupus-like syndrome, which would require drug discontinuation.

Polymorphic ventricular tachycardia or *torsades de pointes*
- Common proarrhythmia associated with Class I or III use.
- Associated with some congenital disorders (Romano–Ward syndrome, Jeville–Lange–Neilson syndrome), concomitant drug therapy (such as tricyclic antidepressants, other Class I and III agents, some macrolide antibiotics and antihistamines) and with electrolyte abnormalities (hypokalaemia, hypomagnesaemia, etc).

Class Ic

Class Ic agents are increasingly used for the management of AF. Indeed, flecainide and propafenone are effective for cardioversion, maintenance of sinus rhythm post-cardioversion and for suppressing paroxysmal AF. These agents are also the drug of choice in patients with the Wolff–Parkinson–White syndrome. The mild beta-blocking properties of propafenone may also help for rate control.

Oral administration seems to be as efficient as the intravenous route and this has led to the 'pill in the pocket' approach to treating paroxysmal AF, where the patient does not take regular drug treatment, but takes one or more oral doses of flecainide or propafenone at the start of a paroxysm of AF, with termination of the arrhythmia in most cases in 8–12 hours. However, this approach should only be used in patients in whom the drug has been shown to be effective, and when the patient is well-informed and compliant with therapy.

Like the Class Ia agents, the major adverse effects associated with Class Ic agents also relate to proarrhythmia. In the Cardiac Arrhythmia Suppression Trial (CAST), flecainide and encainide were used for treating ventricular arrhythmias post-myocardial infarction, with a significant increase in all cause mortality, which was probably due to drug-induced proarrhythmias. However, another overview of flecainide for the treatment of supraventricular tachycardias, where 48% of subjects had structural heart disease, concluded that adverse effects with flecainide were low, although this cannot be equated with safety.

Class I and Class III agents in AF

- Useful for the suppression of paroxysmal AF as well as cardioversion of persistent AF and long-term maintenance of sinus rhythm.
- Class Ic agents (flecainide, propafenone) are relatively safe, effective and commonly used for paroxysmal AF and pharmacological cardioversion.
- Caution is needed in poor left ventricular function and significant ischaemic heart diseases.
- Proarrhythmia may be life threatening, especially in association with electrolyte abnormalities, drugs that prolong the QT interval etc.

Class II antiarrhythmic agents

Beta-blockers have a proven track record in cardiovascular disease, and have many advantages in AF. Contrary to traditional teaching, recent data also support the use of beta-blockers (bisoprolol, carvedilol, metoprolol) in reducing mortality and rehospitalizations in patients with chronic, stable heart failure and left ventricular systolic

dysfunction – thus, these agents should be considered as drugs of choice for rate control in AF patients with chronic heart failure.

Class II agents in AF

- Beta-blockers are useful agents as monotherapy or in combination with digoxin for heart rate control in permanent AF.
- A role to play in maintaining sinus rhythm post-cardioversion and in reducing the paroxysms in paroxysmal AF.
- Beta-blockers are probably the drugs of choice in patients with AF and concomitant ischaemic heart disease, hypertension or chronic stable heart failure.
- A non-specific beta-blocker such as propranolol may also be useful in AF related to thyrotoxicosis.

In acute AF, the use of esmolol, a short- and rapidly acting intravenous beta-blocker, either alone or with digoxin is effective for rate control and can be titrated according to response, and may even cardiovert some patients. Esmolol is also useful in the postoperative setting and post-myocardial infarction, especially with some uncertainty over the use of long-acting beta-blockers in the acute stages.

The side-effects of beta-blockers are well known. Non-selective beta-blockers (eg propranolol) could produce unwanted non-cardiac side-effects, which include bronchospasm and intermittent claudication, as well as (theoretically) reducing the hypoglycaemic symptoms in diabetics. Other side-effects can include lethargy, depression, impotence and sleep disturbance. Cardiac side-effects are mainly due to the negative chronotropic and ionotropic effects, which could potentially worsen heart failure, hypotension and heart block. Sudden cessation of beta-blocker therapy could also (theoretically) result in a 'beta-blocker withdrawal syndrome' with severe hypertension, precipitation of angina/infarction and complications similar to a phaeochromocytoma crisis.

Class III antiarrhythmic agents

Sotalol

Sotalol combines class III activity with non-selective beta-blocking (Class II) activity and is an effective drug in maintaining sinus rhythm postcardioversion and decreasing the paroxysms of AF. At the low doses (under 80 mg daily) commonly used in the UK, Class II effects usually predominate over the class III activity.

Sotalol has been used intravenously (not available in the UK) to cardiovert recent onset AF in patients with good left ventricular function, although oral sotalol is relatively ineffective. Sotalol has the side-effect profile of beta-blockers and importantly, can predispose to proarrhythmia, with life-threatening *torsade de pointes* and ventricular tachycardia in 2% of patients.

Amiodarone

Amiodarone is one of the most widely used antiarrhythmic drugs, especially in patients with underlying ischaemic and/or structural heart disease. Amiodarone, administered both intravenously and orally, appears to be safe and effective for cardioversion of persistent AF. The recent Canadian Trial of Atrial Fibrillation (CTAF) study compared amiodarone with sotalol and propafenone in 403 patients; after 16 months, 63% of patients taking sotalol or propafenone had a recurrence of AF, compared with 35% of those taking amiodarone.

Nevertheless, amiodarone probably has the worst extra-cardiac side-effect profile among all antiarrhythmic drugs, although most of the side-effects are reversible on drug discontinuation. At advanced age, maintenance doses higher than 300 mg/day and pre-existing restrictive lung disease seem to predispose to lung toxicity with amiodarone.

Long-term administration of amiodarone can result in corneal microdeposits, slate grey to bluish discolouration of skin and photosensitivity. Amiodarone also inhibits the peripheral conversion of T4 to T3, resulting in disturbances in thyroid function in approximately 4% of the people, which could manifest in the form of hypothyroidism or hyperthyroidism. Rarely, there is liver damage (which may lead to cirrhosis), interstitial pneumonitis, polyneuropathy and lung fibrosis.

Baseline screening tests before amiodarone use should include thyroid and liver function tests, which should also be monitored during therapy. Slit lamp eye examination may be necessary at times and a chest X-ray is advisable during follow-up.

Amiodarone in AF

- Effective for cardioversion and is the drug of choice in patients with resistant AF and in paroxysmal AF if poor cardiac function is present.
- Oral administration may take weeks to achieve therapeutic concentrations in view of the long half-life ($t_{1/2}$ = 28 days), but intravenous administration of amiodarone has a fast onset of action.
- Intravenous administration should preferably be done via central venous catheter as it may lead to inflammation of the peripheral veins.
- Many side-effects, but most are reversible on drug discontinuation.

Other agents

Dofetilide is a new Class III agent with promising results. In the recent placebo-controlled DIAMOND-CHF study, in patients with symptomatic congestive heart failure and left ventricular dysfunction (a high risk group) where 391 patients had AF, spontaneous cardioversion had occurred in 44% of the dofetilide group compared to 17% of the placebo group after 12 months. Dofetilide was also more effective than placebo in maintaining sinus rhythm. Other Class III agents, such as azimilide, are the subject of ongoing studies and some initial results are encouraging.

Class IV antiarrhythmic agents

The non-dihydropyridine calcium antagonists, verapamil and diltiazem, act on calcium channels, reducing atrioventricular impulse conduction. These rate-limiting calcium antagonists are useful for ventricular rate control in AF when administered orally and intravenously, either as monotherapy or in combination with digoxin. However they are ineffective for the cardioversion of AF and/or for the prevention of paroxysmal AF. The predominant adverse effects of these agents are related to negative ionotropic and chronotropic effects. Toxicity could result in bradycardia, asystole and congestive cardiac failure.

Clonidine

Sympathetic tone is known to play an important role in the genesis and maintenance of AF, as well as in the degree of atrioventricular node conduction and ventricular response. Clonidine, an imidazoline compound, is an agent that decreases discharges in sympathetic preganglionic fibres in the splanchnic nerve and in postganglionic fibres of cardiac nerves, acting directly at α_2-receptors

in the lower brainstem region to suppress sympathetic outflow. Clonidine also stimulates parasympathetic outflow, resulting in prolongation of the refractoriness of the atrioventricular node.

Recent evidence from small clinical trials would suggest that clonidine (eg 0.1 mg orally initially, then 0.1 mg orally at 2 hours if heart rate >100 beats/min) can control the ventricular rate at 6 hours in new-onset AF, with an efficacy comparable to digoxin and verapamil (Figure 7.2).

Are antiarrhythmics all equal in terms of prognosis in AF patients?

The choice of pharmacological therapy for AF depends on a number of factors that include the choice of treatment strategy, the nature of AF (paroxysmal or sustained), underlying ischaemic or structural heart disease, co-morbid conditions, the rapidity with which treatment is indicated, and (of course) patient preference. It is important to remember that these drugs do not abolish the arrhythmia, but merely control or suppress it – this therapeutic goal needs to be made clear to the patient.

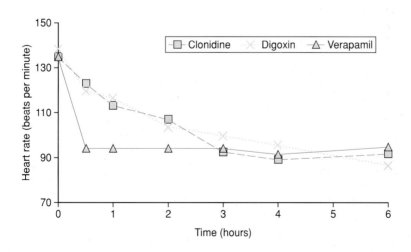

Figure 7.2
Heart rate change over time for patients with atrial fibrillation treated with clonidine, digoxin or verapamil.
Adapted from Simpson CS *et al. Am Heart J* 2001; 142: E3.

For example, digoxin has been predominantly used to control the ventricular rate in fast AF, or in permanent AF, but very often it has been prescribed (erroneously) in other patients with AF, for example, in paroxysmal AF or for cardioversion to sinus rhythm. Indeed, digoxin is no better than placebo in cardioverting AF to sinus rhythm and may even exacerbate paroxysmal AF by increasing the number of paroxysms that tend to occur at faster heart rates.

The effect of antiarrhythmic drugs on mortality in patients with AF is not inconsequential. For example, a report from the Stroke Prevention in Atrial Fibrillation (SPAF) trial found an increase in mortality in patients with AF who were treated with antiarrhythmic drugs (primarily quinidine) if concomitant congestive heart failure was present, with a relative risk for cardiac death of 3.3 and arrhythmic death of 5.8. In the DIAMOND-CHF study, there was a 41% mortality in the dofetilide group compared with 42% in the placebo group, at 18 months. There is no evidence that any antiarrhythmic agent lowers mortality in AF *per se*, although in congestive heart failure, beta-blockers and amiodarone have been shown to have some mortality advantage.

While the presence of AF significantly increases mortality in patients with heart failure, the overall prognosis does seems to be improving in these patients, perhaps reflecting improvements in therapy for heart failure and the avoidance of Class I antiarrhythmic agents.

Sensible prescribing of antiarrhythmic agents is needed. Class I agents should be avoided in patients with heart failure, severe underlying coronary artery disease or other structural heart disease, while digoxin and amiodarone are probably safe. It remains to be seen whether or not the benefits of beta-blockers in patients with congestive heart failure translate to patients with AF.

Drugs for AF and heart failure

Treatment of heart failure in patients with AF has three aspects: prevention of AF in patients with heart failure; treatment of AF to treat the heart failure and treatment of heart failure where continuing AF is present.

Prevention

The issue of drugs for the prevention of *de novo* AF has not been adequately addressed. However, some evidence is available for the ACE inhibitors and dofetilide in patients with myocardial infarction and heart failure respectively. The Danish TRACE study examined the effect of an ACE inhibitor in preventing AF in patients with reduced left ventricular function secondary to acute myocardial infarction: 1,577 patients in sinus rhythm were randomized between trandopril and placebo. After follow-up for between two and four years, 64 patients had developed AF: 42 (5.3%) in the placebo group and 22 (2.8%) in the trandolapril group ($p<0.05$) (RR, 0.45; 95% CI, 0.26-0.76; $p<0.01$). The DIAMOND-CHF study found that dofetilide was more effective than placebo at maintaining sinus rhythm in 1,090 patients with symptomatic congestive heart failure randomized between dofetilide and placebo [11/556 (0.02%) vs 35/534 (0.07%), $p<0.001$].

Treatment of AF in patients with heart failure

AF is commonly associated with heart failure and physicians regularly treat both conditions concurrently. A recent systematic review by Khand *et al* of the management of AF in patients with heart failure found eight studies pertaining to acute AF and 24 pertaining to chronic AF. For patients with acute AF this review concluded that ventricular rate control, anticoagulation and treatment for heart failure should be used simultaneously before cardioversion was attempted. Digoxin was relatively ineffective at controlling ventricular response and for cardioversion, while IV diltiazem was rapidly effective at controlling ventricular rate but had limited evidence suggesting it is safe. Amiodarone controlled ventricular rate rapidly and increased the rate of cardioversion. In chronic AF and heart failure, anticoagulation was essential, although the strategy thereafter was not clear from the evidence: either cardiovert and maintain sinus rhythm with amiodarone, or control ventricular rate combined with anticoagulation.

Brignole *et al* performed a randomized controlled trial of the clinical effects of atrioventricular junction ablation and pacemaker insertion versus conventional drug treatment in 66 patients with chronic (lasting greater than six months) AF who had heart failure and heart rate >90 bpm on three standard ECGs recorded on different days. After 12 months, lower symptom scores were found in the ablation group (28 patients) for both palpitations and dyspnoea versus the drug treatment group (26 patients), but there were no differences seen between the groups on objective measures of cardiac performance (that is, echocardiography and exercise ECG).

The DIAMOND-CHF study found that dofetilide was superior to placebo in converting AF (44% vs 13% at 12 months, $p<0.001$) and preventing its recurrence after cardioversion ($p<0.001$) in patients with heart failure. In another study of 103 patients with AF and congestive heart failure, amiodarone was found to be superior to placebo in converting to sinus rhythm from AF (16/51 vs 4/52, $p=0.002$). Amiodarone may also prevent the new development of AF in heart failure: in CHF-STAT, of the 531 patients in sinus rhythm with CHF, only 11 of 268 patients on amiodarone compared with 22 of the 263 on placebo developed AF ($p=0.005$).

Treatment of heart failure in patients with concurrent AF

The treatment of heart failure is well established with evidence for the use of diuretics, angiotensin-converting enzyme inhibitors, beta-blockers, digoxin and spironolactone. As previously stated, AF and heart failure commonly co-exist and so inevitably trials of various treatments for heart failure have included patients with AF. No evidence was found that sub-groups of patients with concurrent heart failure and AF do not benefit from the validated treatments for heart failure listed.

Table 7.5
Prevalence of AF in relation to NYHA severity of heart failure

Predominant NYHA Type	Prevalence of AF %	Study (year published)
I	4	SOLVD-prevention (1992)
II-III	10–26	SOLVD-treatment (1991)
		CHF-STAT (1995)
		MERIT-HF (1999)
		Diamond (1999)
III-IV	20–29	Middlekauff (1991)
		Stevenson (1996)
		GESICA (1994)
IV	50	CONSENSUS (1987)

NYHA=New York Heart Association; AF=atrial fibrillation; SOLVD=Studies of Left Ventricular Dysfunction; CHF-STAT=Survival Trial of Antiarrhythmic Therapy in Congestive Heart Failure; MERIT-HF=Metoprolol CR/XL Randomized Intervention Trial in Congestive Heart Failure; GESICA=Grupo Estudio de la Sobrevida en la Ensufficienca Cardiaca en Argentina (V); CONSENSUS=Co-operative North Scandinavian Enalapril Survival Study.
Reproduced with permission from Fuster V et al. J Am Coll Cardiol 2001; **38**(4): 1231–66. Copyright 2001 by the American College of Cardiology and the American Heart Association, Inc.

Further reading

Anonymous. Effect of enalapril on mortality and the development of heart failure in asymptomatic patients with reduced left ventricular ejection fractions. The SOLVD Investigators. *N Engl J Med* 1992; **327**: 685–91.

Anonymous. The Cardiac Insufficiency Bisoprolol Study II (CIBIS-II): a randomised trial. *Lancet* 1999; **353**: 9–13.

Brignole M, Menozzi C, Gianfranchi L *et al.* Assessment of atrioventricular junction ablation and VVIR pacemaker versus pharmacological treatment in patients with heart failure and chronic AF: a randomised, controlled study. *Circulation* 1998; **98**: 953–60.

Coplen SE, Antman EM, Berlin JA *et al.* Efficacy and safety of quinidine therapy for maintenance of sinus rhythm after cardioversion: a meta-analysis of RCTs. *Circulation* 1990; **82**: 1106–16.

Conway DSC, Lip GYH. New antiarrhythmic agents for atrial fibrillation. *Curr Opin Invest Drugs* 2001; **2**: 87–92.

Deedwania PC, Singh BN, Ellenbogen K *et al.* Spontaneous conversion and maintenance of sinus rhythm by amiodarone in patients with heart failure and atrial fibrillation: observations from the veterans affairs congestive heart failure survival trial of antiarrhythmic therapy (CHF-STAT). The Department of Veterans Affairs CHF-STAT Investigators. *Circulation* 1998; **98**: 2574–9.

Final consensus statement of the Royal College of Physicians of Edinburgh Consensus Conference on atrial fibrillation in hospital and general practice, 3–4 September 1998. *Br J Haematol* 1999; **104**: 195–6.

Flaker GC, Blackshear JL, McBride R *et al.* Antiarrhythmic drug therapy and cardiac mortality in atrial fibrillation. *J Am Coll Cardiol* 1992; **20**: 527.

Golzari H, Cebul R, Bahler R. Atrial fibrillation: restoration and maintenance of sinus rhythm and indications for anticoagulation therapy. *Ann Intern Med* 1996; **125**: 311–23.

Khand AU, Rankin AC, Kaye GC, Cleland JG. Systematic review of the management of atrial fibrillation in patients with heart failure. *Eur Heart J* 2000; **8**: 614–32.

Li Saw Hee FL, Lip GYH. Digoxin revisited. *Quarterly Journal of Medicine* 1998; **91**: 259–64.

Lip GYH. How would I manage a 60-year-old woman presenting with atrial fibrillation? *Proc R Coll Physicians Edinb* 1999; **29**: 301–6.

Lip GYH, Kamath S. Acute atrial fibrillation. In: Barton SW, ed. *Clinical Evidence*. London: BMJ Publications, 2001: Issue 5.

McNamara RL, Miller MR, Segal JB *et al.* Evidence report on management of new onset atrial fibrillation. Agency of Health Care Policy & Research, US Department of Health and Human Services, 1998.

Murgatroyd FD, Gibson SM, Baiyan X *et al.* Double blind placebo controlled trial of digoxin in symptomatic paroxysmal atrial fibrillation. *Circulation* 1999; **99**: 2765–70.

Pedersen OD, Bagger H, Kober L, Torp-Pedersen C. Trandolapril reduces the incidence of atrial fibrillation after acute myocardial infarction in patients with left ventricular dysfunction. *Circulation* 1999; **100**: 376–80.

Pitt B, Zannad F, Remme WJ *et al.* The effect of spironolactone on morbidity and mortality in patients with severe heart failure. Randomized Aldactone Evaluation Study Investigators. *N Engl J Med* 1999; **341**: 709–17.

Pritchett ELC, Wilkinson WE. Mortality in patients treated with flecainide and encainide for supraventricular arrhythmias. *Am J Cardiol* 1991; **67**: 976–80.

Roy D, Talajic M, Dorian P *et al*, for the Canadian Trial of Atrial Fibrillation Investigators. Amiodarone to prevent recurrence of atrial fibrillation. *N Engl J Med* 2000; **342**: 913–20.

Segal J. Pharmacological interventions for atrial fibrillation (protocol). In: The Cochrane Library, Issue 1, 2000. Oxford: Update Software.

Simpson CS, Ghali WA, Sanfilippo A *et al.* Clinical assessment of clonidine in the treatment of new-onset rapid atrial fibrillation: A prospective, randomized clinical trial. *Am Heart J* 2001; **142**: e3.

Southworth MR, Zarembski D, Viana M, Bauman J. Comparison of sotalol versus quinidine for maintenance of normal sinus rhythm in patients with chronic atrial fibrillation. *Am J Cardiol* 1999; **83** :1629–32.

Stevenson WG, Stevenson LW, Middlekauff HR *et al.* Improving survival for patients with atrial fibrillation and advanced heart failure. *J Am Coll Cardiol* 1996; **28**: 1458–63.

Torp-Pedersen C, Moller M, Bloch-Thomsen PE *et al.* Dofetilide in patients with congestive heart failure and left ventricular dysfunction. *N Engl J Med* 1999; **341**: 857–65.

Zarembski DG, Nolan PE Jr, Slack MK, Caruso AC. Treatment of resistant atrial fibrillation: a meta-analysis comparing amiodarone and flecaininde. *Arch Intern Med* 1995; **155**: 1885–91.

8. Management strategies

Acute atrial fibrillation
Paroxysmal (recurrent) atrial fibrillation
Persistent atrial fibrillation
Permanent atrial fibrillation
Can intervention be worse than non-intervention

One proposed clinical definition of atrial fibrillation (AF) divides patients into acute-onset and chronic AF; the latter are further divided into paroxysmal and sustained. Sustained AF is further divided into persistent and permanent AF (the so-called '3P classification', Figure 8.1).

The differentiation between these clinical categories is dependent upon the history given by the patient, ECG documentation of the current episode and the duration of the last episode of AF. Although this classification is helpful, there is considerable inter- and intra-patient variability in the temporal pattern of AF episodes and therapy must be individualized.

Definitions
- The term 'acute AF' is used to describe either an episode of AF related to a transient and reversible cause or the first onset of AF.
- Paroxysmal (recurrent) AF refers to recurrent, intermittent episodes of AF.
- Persistent AF is sustained AF that can be successfully cardioverted.
- Permanent AF is sustained AF that is either resistant to or not appropriate for cardioversion.

The objectives of management of the patient with AF are largely dependent upon the type of patient, whether or not paroxysmal, persistent or permanent.

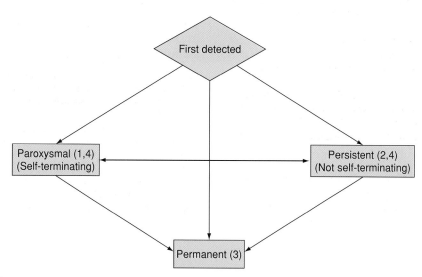

Figure 8.1
Patterns of atrial fibrillation: 1=episodes that generally last less than or equal to seven days (most less than 24 hours); 2=usually more than seven days; 3=cardioversion failed or not attempted; 4=either paroxysmal or persistent AF may be recurrent. Adapted from Fuster V *et al. J Am Coll Cardiol* 2001; **38**(4): 1231–66.

Management approach to AF

- First, is the diagnosis of AF certain?
- Is it paroxysmal or sustained AF, in view of the important management differences between the two conditions? If sustained AF, is it persistent AF or permanent AF?
- Why did the patient develop AF? A search for the underlying aetiological or predisposing factor(s) should be undertaken.
- In acute presentations of AF, the presence of 'acute' precipitating factors (for example, infection) and any complications should be sought.

Acute atrial fibrillation

Evaluation of the cause or precipitating factor for acute AF may be as important as treating the arrhythmia. For example, rendering the patient euthyroid in the context of thyrotoxic AF often results in spontaneous conversion to sinus rhythm in a high proportion of patients. Many patients with alcohol-induced AF will spontaneously revert to sinus rhythm in 24 hours, without the need for cardioversion.

Patients who present with an acute onset of AF should be treated with immediate direct current cardioversion under general anaesthetic, if AF is associated with significant haemodynamic compromise.

Patients who present with acute-onset AF who are haemodynamically stable and asymptomatic, or if they present later than 48 hours after the onset, can initially be treated with a strategy of heart rate control and anticoagulation, as an alternative to cardioversion, allowing time for assessment and evaluation of the patient. In either case effective anticoagulation in the form of heparin and/or warfarin should be initiated to decrease the risk of thromboembolic complications. Associated complications should be managed accordingly, for example, acute heart failure should be treated with diuretics.

Paroxysmal (recurrent) atrial fibrillation

The objectives of management of paroxysmal AF are the suppression of paroxysms and the long-term maintenance of sinus rhythm, as well as appropriate thromboprophylaxis. Many patients with paroxysmal AF are young and 'lone AF' is more common when compared to sustained AF. If a patient is experiencing only mild and infrequent symptoms, it may be possible to avoid antiarrhythmic drugs and their potential for toxicity.

Aims of management in paroxysmal AF

- To control symptoms due to paroxysms of AF
- To minimize haemodynamic sequelae due to paroxysms of AF
- To prevent thromboembolic complications

Where relevant, general measures should always be considered, for example, the withdrawal of caffeine or alcohol if these have been identified as precipitants, and consideration of associated conditions which may benefit from atrial pacing, for example, sick sinus syndrome.

Many patients with paroxysmal AF will have asymptomatic paroxysms, but there is increasing evidence that frequent, uncontrolled paroxysms of fast AF may lead to impairment of cardiac function (the so-called 'tachycardia-induced cardiomyopathy') and a higher progression to sustained AF.

Class I and Class III antiarrhythmic drugs are appropriate choices for patients with paroxysmal AF. For example, flecainide and propafenone (both Class Ic agents) are drugs of first choice in paroxysmal AF, in the absence of contraindications. However, Class I agents should be avoided in the patients with poor cardiac function. Sotalol combines both Class II (beta blockade) and Class III antiarrhythmic effects, although at the low doses commonly used, much of its activity is likely to be related to its beta-blocking activity. Thus, commonly used beta-blockers, such as atenolol or metoprolol, have been used as alternatives to sotalol, especially if paroxysmal AF is related to an adrenergic stimulus (stress, exercise, alcohol, etc), thus avoiding the potential toxicity associated with sotalol. The rate-limiting calcium channel blockers (diltiazem, verapamil) and beta-blockers may help control ventricular rate in paroxysmal AF but may not alter the frequency of episodes. Amiodarone has potentially serious, albeit relatively rare, side-effects but is of value in paroxysmal AF refractory to other measures, the elderly and those with poor left ventricular function. In paroxysmal AF, low doses may be effective with little risk of side-effects or proarrhythmia.

Digoxin should be avoided in paroxysmal AF as this drug makes paroxysmal AF worse. Retrospective analyses have suggested that paroxysms of AF are more frequent and last longer, and the initial heart rate appears no better controlled, whether or not digoxin is being taken. One recent double-blind placebo-controlled trial of digoxin in symptomatic paroxysmal AF found a small effect in reducing the frequency of symptomatic AF episodes, probably due to a reduction in ventricular rate or irregularity rather than an antiarrhythmic action.

Antithrombotic therapy should be considered in patients with paroxysmal AF, since patients with paroxysmal AF have a similar stroke risk to patients with sustained AF, especially in the presence of risk factors. There have been no definitive trials looking specifically at the benefits of antithrombotic therapy in patients with paroxysmal AF *per se* and the range of thromboembolic risk in such patients is likely to be wide. It would seem reasonable to consider antithrombotic therapy based on patients' co-morbidity, age and the presence of structural heart disease.

Persistent atrial fibrillation

In persistent AF, the management objective for patients is cardioversion. The main factor determining the likelihood of successful cardioversion is the duration of AF. Nevertheless, if the underlying aetiology or trigger (eg thyrotoxicosis, chest infection, etc) continues to exert an effect in the patient with persistent AF, attempts at cardioversion may be unsuccessful. Conversely, treatment of the precipitating factor may result in spontaneous reversion to sinus rhythm or increase the chances of successful cardioversion. Persistent AF can be related to paroxysmal AF, where an episode lasts more than 48 hours and spontaneous conversion to sinus rhythm does not occur; that time window presents the duration beyond which formal anticoagulation should be administered before cardioversion.

Cardioversion of persistent AF

- Most patients with recent onset AF, in the absence of structural heart disease and where a precipitant has been corrected, should be considered for cardioversion.
- If AF duration is greater than 48 hours, anticoagulation pre- and post-cardioversion should be considered (see page 56).
- Cardioversion can be performed using a synchronized DC shock or by pharmacological means (Class I or III).

Potential benefits from cardioversion of AF to sinus rhythm

- Improved haemodynamics at rest and with exercise
- Improvement of symptoms
- Possible reduction in the risk of stroke and the need for anticoagulation

---

Predictors of refractoriness to cardioversion or unsuccessful long-term maintenance of sinus rhythm

- Age
- Duration of arrhythmia
- Presence of uncontrolled hypertension
- Structural heart disease
- Presence of other systemic diseases

The duration of AF is probably the most important predictor of successful cardioversion and long-term maintenance of sinus rhythm.

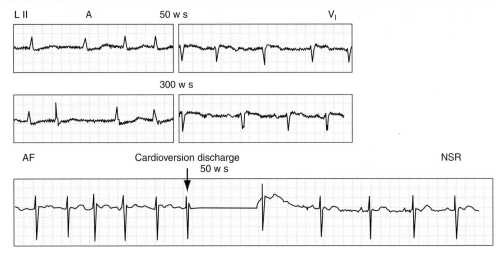

Figure 8.2
Electrical cardioversion of persistent atrial fibrillation.

Methods of cardioversion

Cardioversion may be performed by electrical or pharmacological methods. Meta-analysis of trials that have used pharmacological conversion in conjunction with DC cardioversion provide no evidence that such a strategy leads to a higher initial conversion rate than DC cardioversion alone. While there is a high initial success rate, there is also a significant relapse rate. For example, in the control groups of trials evaluating the role of quinidine in maintaining sinus rhythm after electrical cardioversion, after 12 months only 19–30% of patients were still in sinus rhythm.

Duration of AF is the strongest predictor of failure of conversion (electrical or pharmacological) to and maintenance of sinus rhythm. Lack of response to treatment is also associated with increasing age, the presence of structural heart disease and ongoing precipitant/contributor to AF.

External electrical cardioversion (Figure 8.2), using a synchronised DC shock under a light general anaesthetic, is effective in restoring sinus rhythm. The recommended initial energy for electrical cardioversion is 200 joules and >75% of patients are successfully cardioverted with this energy. Higher energies

(300–360 joules) are needed if 200 joules shocks are unsuccessful in restoring sinus rhythm. The efficacy of electrical cardioversion can be influenced by the underlying aetiology, ranging from 20–90%. The highest recorded success rates for cardioversion are seen in (treated) patients with AF secondary to hyperthyroidism, while the lowest rates are seen in patients with severe mitral regurgitation.

An alternative to electrical cardioversion is pharmacological cardioversion (Table 8.1) to restore and to maintain sinus rhythm and to control the ventricular rate in AF. A Cochrane systematic review is currently in preparation to address these issues. In general, drugs that are usually used for paroxysmal AF or to maintain sinus rhythm after electrical cardioversion are also effective for pharmacological cardioversion, such as the Class I and III agents (Tables 8.2–8.4). In trials that have compared antiarrhythmic agents to controls, a systematic review reported that quinidine, flecainide, propafenone, amiodarone, and ibutilide/dofetilide were all effective. However, there were insufficient data on disopyramide, and sotalol was shown to be ineffective. Digoxin is ineffective in restoring sinus rhythm, with or without the presence of heart failure.

Maintenance of sinus rhythm

Many of the trials investigating the role of antiarrhythmic agents for the maintenance of sinus rhythm have been limited by small numbers and variable quality of study methodology. Nevertheless, the systematic review by McNamara *et al* concluded that there was strong evidence for the efficacy of quinidine, disopyramide, flecainide, propafenone and sotalol for maintaining sinus rhythm after DC cardioversion. Zarembski *et al* performed a meta-analysis of trials that

Table 8.1
Recommendations for pharmacological cardioversion of atrial fibrillation of (a) less than or equal to seven days' duration (b) more than seven days' duration

(a)

Drug	Route of administration	Type of recommendation	Level of evidence
Agents with proven efficacy			
Dofetilide	Oral	I	A
Flecainide	Oral or intravenous	I	A
Ibutilide	Intravenous	I	A
Propafenone	Oral or intravenous	I	A
Amiodarone	Oral or intravenous	IIa	A
Quinidine	Oral	IIb	B
Less effective/incompletely studied agents			
Procainamide	Intravenous	IIb	C
Digoxin	Oral or intravenous	III	A
Sotalol	Oral or intravenous	III	A

(b)

Drug	Route of administration	Type of recommendation	Level of evidence
Agents proven effective			
Dofetilide	Oral	I	A
Amiodarone	Oral or intravenous	IIa	A
Ibutilide	Intravenous	IIa	A
Flecainide	Oral	IIb	B
Propafenone	Oral or intravenous	IIb	B
Quinidine	Oral	IIb	B
Less effective/incompletely studied agents			
Procainamide	Intravenous	IIb	C
Sotalol	Oral or intravenous	III	A
Digoxin	Oral or intravenous	III	C

Adapted from Fuster V *et al. J Am Coll Cardiol* 2001; **38**(4): 1231–65. Copyright 2001 by the American College of Cardiology and the American Heart Association, Inc.

Level of evidence=highest (A) evidence derived from multiple randomized clinical trials; intermediate (B) derived from limited number of randomized trials, nonrandomized studies or observational registries; lowest (C) derived from expert consensus only. Type of recommendation: Class I=conditions for which there is evidence for and/or agreement that treatment/procedure is useful and effective; Class II=conditions for which there is conflicting evidence and/or divergent opinion on usefulness/effectiveness of treatment/procedure – Class IIa evidence is in favour of treatment/procedure, Class IIb usefulness/efficacy is less well established; Class III conditions for which evidence and opinion suggest treatment/procedure is not useful/effective and may be harmful in some cases.

Table 8.2

Recommended doses of drugs proven effective for pharmacological cardioversion of atrial fibrillation.

Drug*	Route of administration	Dosage**		Potential adverse effects
Amiodarone	Oral	Inpatient: 1.2–1.8 g per day in divided dose until 10 g, then 200–400 mg per day maintenance or 30 mg/kg as single dose		Hypotension, bradycardia, QT prolongation, torsade de pointes (rare), GI upset, constipation, phlebitis (IV)
		Outpatient: 600–800 mg per day divided dose until 10 g total, then 200–400 mg per day maintenance		
	Intravenous/oral	5–7 mg/kg over 30–60 min, then 1.2–1.8 g per day continuous IV or in divided oral doses until 10 g total, then 200–400 mg per day maintenance		
Dofetilide	Oral	Creatinine clearance (ml/min)	Dose (μg BID)	QT prolongation, torsade de pointes; adjust dose for renal function, body size and age
		>60	500	
		40–60	250	
		20–40	125	
		<20	Contraindicted	
Flecainide	Oral	200–300 mg†		Hypotension, rapidly conducting atrial flutter
	Intravenous	1.5–3.0 mg/kg over 10–20 min†		
Ibutilide	Intravenous	1 mg over 10 min; repeat 1 mg when necessary		QT prolongation, torsade de pointes
Propafenone	Oral	450–600 mg		Hypotension, rapidly conducting atrial flutter
	Intravenous	1.5–2.0 mg/kg over 10–20 min†		
Quinidine‡	Oral	0.75–1.5 g in divided doses over 6–12 h, usually with a rate-slowing drug		QT prolongation, torsade de pointes, GI upset, hypotension

GI=gastrointestinal; IV=intravenous; BID=twice a day

*Drugs are listed alphabetically; **Best to consult datasheet for dosaging regimes; †Insufficient data are available on which to base specific recommendations for the use of one loading regimen over another for patients with ischaemic heart disease or impaired left ventricular function, and these drugs should be used cautiously or not at all in such patients. ‡The use of quinidine loading to achieve pharmacological conversion of atrial fibrillation is controversial, and safer methods are available with the alternative agents listed in the table.

Reproduced with permission from Fuster V et al. J Am Coll Cardiol 2001; **38**(4): 1231–65. Copyright 2001 by the American College of Cardiology and the American Heart Association, Inc.

included amiodarone or flecainide in the treatment of chronic (ie more than two weeks' duration) AF. They found six trials of amiodarone (315 patients) and two of flecainide (163 patients). In both the flecainide studies, treatment was preceded by DC cardioversion, and in the amiodarone trials, DC cardioversion was used if amiodarone did not induce sinus rhythm. Indirect comparison suggested that amiodarone was more effective at maintaining sinus rhythm up to one year.

Table 8.3

Typical doses of drugs used to maintain sinus rhythm in patients with atrial fibrillation*

Drug	Daily dosage	Potential adverse effects
Amiodarone†	100–400 mg	Photosensitivity, pulmonary toxicity, polyneuropathy, GI upset, bradycardia, torsade de pointes (rare), hepatic toxicity, thyroid dysfunction
Disopyramide	400–750 mg	Torsade de pointes, HF, glaucoma, urinary retention, dry mouth
Dofetilide‡	500–1000 mg	Torsade de pointes
Flecainide	200–300 mg	Ventricular tachycardia, congestive HF, enhanced AV nodal conduction (conversion to atrial flutter)
Procainamide	1000–4000 mg	Torsade de pointes, lupus-like syndrome, GI symptoms
Propafenone	450–900 mg	Ventricular tachycardia, congestive HF, enhanced AV nodal conduction (conversion to atrial flutter)
Quinidine	600–1500 mg	Torsade de pointes, GI upset, enhanced AV nodal conduction
Sotalol‡	240–320 mg	Torsade de pointes, congestive HF, brachycardia, exacerbation of chronic obstructuve or bronchospastic lung disease

GI=gastrointestinal; AV=atrioventricular; HF=heart failure.

*Drugs and doses given are based on published studies; †a loading dose of 600 mg per day is usually given for one month or 1000 mg per day over one week; ‡dose should be adjusted for renal function and QT-interval response during in-hospital initiation phase.

Reproduced with permission from Fuster V *et al. J Am Coll Cardiol* 2001; **38**(4): 1231–65. Copyright 2001 by the American College of Cardiology and the American Heart Association, Inc.

Recommendations for anticoagulation for cardioversion of AF

- The administration of warfarin for three weeks before elective cardioversion of AF of <48 hours' duration; continuation of warfarin therapy for a minimum of four weeks after cardioversion.
- Administration of intravenous heparin followed by warfarin if cardioversion cannot be postponed for three weeks.
- Treat atrial flutter similarly.
- No anticoagulant therapy for SVT or AF of <48 hours' duration.
- In 'high risk' individuals, consideration should be given towards continuing anticoagulation therapy in view of the risk of thrombo-embolism if AF recurs.

Based on the 6th ACCP Consensus Conference on Antithrombotic Therapy [Chest 2001].

Antithrombotic therapy for cardioversion

In patients with persistent AF, appropriate use of antiarrhythmic therapy to maintain sinus rhythm and anticoagulation to reduce the risk of thromboembolism post-cardioversion should be considered.

Transoesophageal echocardiography guided cardioversion

In an attempt to simplify and minimize the anticoagulation regime required for cardioversion, transoesophageal echocardiography (TEE)-guided cardioversion is a new strategy, where the patient is heparinized and warfarin initiated (target INR 2.0–3.0), following which biplane or multiplane TEE is performed to assess left atrial size and to check for the presence of atrial thrombi or possible mitral stenosis.

If no thrombus or other adverse features (spontaneous echocontrast, valve disease, etc) are seen, cardioversion is then performed, and warfarin continued for a minimum of four weeks. If thrombus is seen, severe spontaneous echo contrast is present, the left atrial appendage cannot be adequately evaluated for technical reasons, or TEE is contraindicated, patients receive four weeks of warfarin before elective cardioversion, as per conventional management.

Cardioversion versus rate control

Cardioversion of AF has been shown to improve cardiac haemodynamics and quality of life in the short term. The potential benefits of a return to sinus rhythm include an improvement in patient wellbeing, improved haemodynamic status and exercise capability (secondary to the return of atrial filling, and consequent improved cardiac output), the avoidance of (potentially dangerous) drug therapy and perhaps a reduction in stroke and thromboembolic risk. Indeed, there is consistently an improvement in exercise capacity and left ventricular function following a return to sinus rhythm. The return of atrial systole can contribute as much as 30% of the stroke volume, especially in the elderly and in patients with evidence of diastolic dysfunction. The return of atrial transport also reduces atrial size and stasis in the atria, thus potentially reducing the risk of stroke and thromboembolism.

There is a paucity of data comparing whether or not a strategy of rate control is superior to a strategy of aggressive cardioversion ('rhythm control') with respect to long-term mortality and morbidity. The superiority of a strategy of heart rate control and antithrombotic therapy ('rate control') over a strategy of aggressive cardioversion ('rhythm control') is still unproven, and is being tested in several large randomized trials.

Permanent atrial fibrillation

In permanent AF the arrhythmia has been present for a long time and that cardioversion has not been indicated or that one or several attempts of cardioversion has failed to restore sinus rhythm. The objectives of management in such patients are therefore heart rate control and antithrombotic therapy. Heart rate control can be achieved by pharmacological and non-pharmacological methods.

The systematic review by McNamara et al identified 45 trials evaluating 17 different agents for rate control in AF, and concluded that the calcium channel blockers dilitiazem and verapamil were more effective than placebo or digoxin in reducing heart rate at rest and during exercise. Beta-blockers also reduced heart rate during rest and exercise, but were associated with reduced exercise tolerance in a number of studies. In this overview, the evidence on digoxin was inconclusive.

Digoxin is commonly used for heart rate control, but is less likely to control the ventricular rate during pyrexia, stress, exercise (when vagal tone is low and sympathetic tone is high) etc. It also has little or no ability to terminate the arrhythmia or to maintain sinus rhythm post-cardioversion. The onset of rate control with digoxin is often delayed for several hours, even with intravenous therapy and this slow onset of action may be undesirable in acute situations. Many patients given digoxin usually require the addition of a beta-blocker or a rate-limiting calcium channel blocker for optimal rate control.

The role of antithrombotic therapy in patients with AF has been well established in recent clinical trials, and is discussed further in chapter 9.

Table 8.4
Pharmacological agents for heart rate control in patients with atrial fibrillation

Intravenous agents

Drug*	Loading dose	Onset	Maintenance dose	Major side-effects	Class recommendation
Diltiazem	0.25 mg/kg IV over 2 min	2–7 min	5–15 mg per hour infusion	Hypotension, heart block, HF	I†
Esmolol‡	0.5 mg/kg over 1 min	5 min	0.05–0.2 mg/kg/min	Hypotension, heart block, brachycardia, asthma, HF	I
Metoprolol‡	2.5–5 mg IV bolus over 2 min; up to 3 doses	5 min	N/A	Hypotension, heart block, brachycardia, asthma, HF	I†
Propranolol†	0.15 mg/kg IV	5 min	N/A	Hypotension, heart block, brachycardia, asthma, HF	I†
Verapamil	0.075–0.15 mg/kg IV over 2 min	3–5 min	N/A	Hypotension, heart block, HF	I†
Digoxin	0.25 mg IV each 2 h, up to 1.5 mg	2 h	0.125–0.25 mg daily	Digitalis toxicity, heart block, brachycardia	IIb**

Oral agents

Drug*	Loading dose	Onset	Maintenance dose	Major side-effects	Class recommendation
Digoxin	0.25 mg PO each 2 h; up to 1.5 mg	2 h	0.125–0.375 mg daily	Digitalis toxicity, heart block, brachycardia	I
Diltiazem	N/A	2–4 h	120–360 mg daily in divided doses; slow release available	Hypotension, heart block, HF	I
Metoprolol†	N/A	4–6 h	25–100 mg BID	Hypotension, heart block, brachycardia, asthma, HF	I
Propranolol†	N/A	60–90 min	80–240 mg daily in divided doses	Hypotension, heart block, brachycardia, asthma, HF	I
Verapamil	N/A	1–2 h	120–360 mg daily in divided doses; slow release available	Hypotension, heart block, HF, digoxin interaction	I
Amiodarone	800 mg daily for 1 week; 600 mg daily for 1 week; 400 mg daily for 4–6 week	1–3 week	200 mg daily	Pulmonary toxicity, skin discolouration, hyperthyroidism, corneal deposits, optic neuropathy, warfarin interaction, proarryhthmia	IIb

HF=heart failure.

*Drugs are listed alphabetically within each class of recommendation; **Type I in congestive HF; †Type IIb in congestive HF; ‡only representative members of the type of beta-adrenergic antagonist drugs are included in the table. See Table 8.1 for explanation of Type recommendation.

Reproduced with permission from Fuster V et al. J Am Coll Cardiol 2001; **38**(4): 1231–65). Copyright 2001 by the American College of Cardiology and the American Heart Association, Inc.

Strategies in permanent AF

- Heart rate control should be achieved using digoxin, beta-blockers, non-dihydropyridine calcium antagonists (verapamil or diltiazem), or combinations, as appropriate.

- Thromboprophylaxis is essential, and warfarin or aspirin used according to risk stratification criteria.

- If medical therapy for rate control fails, consider non-pharmacological measures.

- Remember the need for permanent pacemakers in symptomatic bradycardias and chronotrophic incompetence (that is, inappropriate increase in heart rate in response to exercise/exertion).

Can intervention be worse than non-intervention

The '3P classification' (that is, paroxysmal, persistent and permanent) allows adequate division along the lines of clinical objectives of management and can assist management strategies by defining treatment objectives, although many patients change from one category to another and therapy must be individualized (see inside front-cover flowchart). However, intervention can occasionally be worse than non-intervention, in view of the associated morbidity (and occasional mortality) by the use of antiarrhythmic and antithrombotic agents.

For example, care should be employed when interpreting the results of the clinical trials, which demonstrate unequivocal benefit of anticoagulation in AF. These trials were conducted on a carefully selected patient population and where anticoagulation was strictly monitored in well-motivated investigators and patients, who essentially received careful follow-up and 'packages of care'. Whether or not these results could be fully extrapolated to general clinical practice is not entirely clear. In patients taking antithrombotic therapy, the annual risks of intracranial haemorrhage increase from 0.1% in controls to 0.3% in warfarin groups in the pooled analysis of the AF Investigators, which represents an excess of two intracranial bleeds per annum per thousand patients treated. The bleeding risk with anticoagulation was particularly associated with an INR greater than 3.0, fluctuating INRs and with uncontrolled hypertension.

As previously mentioned, the inappropriate use of antiarrhythmic drugs could lead to unwanted consequences including proarrhythmia and death, and hence these drugs have to be used with great caution after adequate consideration of the risk and benefits of the drug in the individual patient. Antiarrhythmic agents that reduce mortality include amiodarone and beta-blockers, although this evidence is based on trials of treatment of congestive heart failure, rather than in AF *per se*. Indeed, the vast majority of these patients will have been in sinus rhythm. There is no evidence that any of the other antiarrhythmic agents lower mortality in AF. There is some evidence that some are associated with increased mortality.

These caveats of intervention have to be weighed against the substantial increase in risk of stroke and thromboembolism associated with AF without antithrombotic therapy use, as well as heart failure and other haemodynamic consequences of poor heart rate or AF rhythm control.

Further reading

Amiodarone Trials Meta-analysis Investigators. Effect of prophylactic amiodarone on mortality after acute myocardial infarction and in congestive heart failure: meta-analysis of individual data from 6500 patients in randomised trials. *Lancet* 1997; **350**: 1417–24.

Bonet S, Agusti A, Arnau J *et al*. Beta-blocking agents in heart failure: a meta-analysis of clinical trials. *Arch Intern Med* 2000; **160**: 621–27.

Coplen SE, Antman EM, Berlin JA *et al*. Efficacy and safety of quinidine therapy for maintenance of sinus rhythm after cardioversion: a meta-analysis of RCTs. *Circulation* 1990; **82**: 1106–16.

Golzari H, Cebul R, Bahler R. Atrial fibrillation: restoration and maintenance of sinus rhythm and indications for anticoagulation therapy. *Ann Intern Med* 1996; **125**: 311–23.

Farshi R, Kistner D, Sarma JSM *et al*. Ventricular rate control in chronic atrial fibrillation during daily activity and programmed exercise: A cross-over open label study of five drug regimens. *J Am Coll Cardiol* 1999; **33**: 304–10.

Final consensus statement of the Royal College of Physicians of Edinburgh Consensus Conference on atrial fibrillation in hospital and general practice, 3-4 September 1998. *Br J Haematol* 1999; **104**: 195–6.

Fuster V, Ryden LE, Asinger RW *et al*. ACC/AHA/ESC guidelines for the management of patients with atrial fibrillation: executive summary. *J Am Coll Cardiol* 2001; **38**(4): 1231–65.

Golzari H, Cebul R, Bahler R. Atrial fibrillation: restoration and maintenance of sinus rhythm and indications for anticoagulation therapy. *Ann Intern Med* 1996; **125**: 311–23.

Lip GYH. How would I manage a 60-year-old woman presenting with atrial fibrillation? *Proc R Coll Phys Edinb* 1999; **29**: 301–6.

McNamara RL, Miller MR, Segal JB *et al*. Evidence report on management of new onset atrial fibrillation. Agency of Health Care Policy & Research, US Department of Health and Human Services, 1998.

Murgatroyd FD, Gibson SM, Baiyan X *et al*. Double blind placebo controlled trial of digoxin in symptomatic paroxysmal atrial fibrillation. *Circulation* 1999; **99**: 2765–70.

Rawles JM, Metcalfe MJ, Jennings K. Time of occurrence, duration, and ventricular rate of paroxysmal atrial fibrillation: the effect of digoxin. *Br Heart J* 1990; **63**: 225–7.

Segal J. Pharmacological interventions for atrial fibrillation (protocol). In: The Cochrane Library, Issue 1, 2000. Oxford: Update Software.

Southworth MR, Zarembski D, Viana M, Bauman J. Comparison of sotalol versus quinidine for maintenance of normal sinus rhythm in patients with chronic atrial fibrillation. *Am J Cardiol* 1999; **83**: 1629–32.

Torp-Pedersen C, Moller M, Bloch-Thomsen PE *et al*. Dofetilide in patients with congestive heart failure and left ventricular dysfunction. *N Engl J Med* 1999; **341**: 857–65.

Zarembski DG, Nolan PE Jr, Slack MK, Caruso AC. Treatment of resistant atrial fibrillation: a meta-analysis comparing amiodarone and flecaininde. *Arch Intern Med* 1995; **155**: 1885–91.

9. Antithrombotic therapy

Antithrombotic therapy for atrial fibrillation in the clinical setting
Acute atrial fibrillation
Persistent atrial fibrillation
Paroxysmal and permanent atrial fibrillation
Atrial fibrillation patients presenting with stroke
Risk stratification
Bleeding risks
Other strategies in providing thromboprophylaxis
From trials to clinical practice

Antithrombotic therapy for atrial fibrillation in the clinical setting

Atrial fibrillation (AF) is the most common cardiac disorder leading to stroke and thromboembolism. Most of the stroke and thromboembolic events in patients with AF are due to thrombus formation in the fibrillating left atria. The loss of atrial systole and increased atrial stasis (visualized as the phenomenon of spontaneous echocontrast using transoesophageal echocardiography), in association with abnormalities of haemostasis and platelet activation in AF all predispose to thrombus formation (thrombogenesis). Risk factors for stroke, such as valve disease, hypertension and heart failure, are additive to the risk associated with AF *per se*.

The presence of non-valvular AF increases the risk of stroke approximately five-fold. The importance of AF as a risk factor for stroke increases with age, with an attributable risk for stroke at the age of 50–59 years of 1.5% and at 80–89 years, a risk of 23.5%. AF is usually present in about 15–20% of patients with acute stroke, and is associated with a 1.5 to 3.0-fold higher mortality than that for stroke patients who are in sinus rhythm. Strokes attributed to AF also tend to be more severe, with greater disability, longer hospital stay and lower rate of discharge to the patient's own home. There is also a high recurrence rate and silent cerebral infarcts frequently occur. The provision of thromboprophylaxis in AF can be described in three main clinical settings.

The provision of thromboprophylaxis in AF
- Use of heparin in acute AF
- Warfarin for cardioversion of persistent AF
- Aspirin or warfarin as long-term prophylaxis in paroxysmal or permanent AF

Acute atrial fibrillation

In patients presenting *de novo* with AF, a clear history of arrhythmia onset is often necessary. If the duration of AF is clearly less than 48 hours, cardioversion may be performed without the need for long-term anticoagulation post-cardioversion, although there are no randomized trials specifically answering this question. Nevertheless, intra-atrial thrombus has been detected by transoesophageal echocardiography in approximately 15% of patients presenting with an acute onset (<48 hours) AF, although the possibility remains that many of these patients had earlier developed AF asymptomatically. Thus, in cases of uncertainty, anticoagulation is warranted.

In summary, patients presenting *de novo* with AF should be started on intravenous heparin following initial diagnosis, achieving an activated partial thromboplastin time (APPT) ratio of 2–3, which should reduce the risk of thrombus formation.

Heparin

The prime role of heparin in AF is when immediate anticoagulation is desired until adequate INR is attained with warfarin or patient needs to undergo urgent cardioversion. Therapy is administered by an intravenous infusion and monitored by measurement of the APTT, which is sensitive to the levels of thrombin, factor Xa, and factor IXa. The therapeutic range of APTT depends on the commercial reagent used to measure it. But on average, a ratio of >1.5 has a therapeutic effect. The dose of heparin needed to maintain APTT in a therapeutic range varies widely and different methods of deciding the right dose for the patient have been proposed. These include dose-adjustment nomograms, weight-adjusted nomograms, and computer algorithms.

Recently, low molecular weight heparin (LMWH) preparations, which are administered subcutaneously and act by facilitating the inhibition of coagulation factor Xa by antithrombin, have been introduced with good results in AF. LMWH does not require monitoring by measurement of the APPT, and its ease of administration has resulted in its increasing use in place of the traditional unfractionated heparin infusion.

Persistent atrial fibrillation

In cases where the duration of AF is >48 hours, anticoagulation with warfarin (INR 2–3) should be started for a minimum of three weeks, and if appropriate, cardioversion should be attempted and anticoagulation continued for at least four weeks. Recommendations from the American College of Chest Physicians regarding anticoagulation for cardioversion of AF were summarized earlier in chapter 8.

Recently, transoesophageal echocardiography has evolved as an attractive alternative to prolonged anticoagulation before DC cardioversion. The use of transoesophageal echocardiography may allow cardioversion to be done earlier, minimizing the risk for embolism with a shorter anticoagulation period, and may be associated with less clinical instability than conventional therapy.

Paroxysmal and permanent atrial fibrillation

In a recent meta-analysis of antithrombotic therapy in AF, the use of anticoagulation in AF has been shown to reduce the risk of stroke by 62% [95% confidence intervals (CI) 48–72%], while aspirin reduces the risk by 22% (CI, 2–38%). Absolute risk reductions with warfarin were 1.5% per year for primary prevention and 2.5% per year for secondary prevention. Furthermore, adjusted dose warfarin reduced the risk by 36% (CI, 14–52%) relative to aspirin. Other systematic reviews, including Cochrane reviews, have reached the same conclusions. However, a recent systematic review by Taylor et al based on endpoints of vascular death, found a non-significant 14% reduction in fatal endpoints when warfarin was compared to antiplatelet therapy.

Recent trials carried out in primary care have failed to demonstrate significant benefits of warfarin therapy, but the AFASAK2 trial had been stopped early (thus underpowered) and the PATAF study has been criticized for methodology problems.

In the pooled meta-analysis by the AF investigators of the five initial primary prevention trials, an annual rate of all strokes of 4.5% was found in the control group and a rate of 1.4% in the warfarin group, representing an overall risk reduction of 68% (95% confidence intervals 50–79%). Warfarin prophylaxis also resulted in a similar risk reduction in stroke with residual deficit, a decrease in mortality of 33%, and a decrease in the combined adverse outcome (stroke, systemic embolism or death) of 48%. Warfarin usage was particularly beneficial as secondary prevention in the EAFT study, where the risk of stroke was reduced from 12% to 4% per year (Hazard ratio: 0.34; 95% CI: 0.20–0.57).

Analyses of the optimal anticoagulation intensity for stroke prevention in AF demonstrated that stroke risk appeared to be substantially increased at INR levels <2.0. The inr was a powerful and independent determinant of the risk of stroke, and when compared with patients with an INR of 2.0, those with an INR of 1.7 had a two-fold increase in the risk of stroke. At INRs >3.0, the risk of haemorrhage increases exponentially. Thus, the optimal INR range for thromboprophylaxis in non-valvular AF should be 2.0–3.0 (see Figure 9.1).

Despite the impressive figures derived from the trials, the optimal efficacy of warfarin prophylaxis is probably underestimated, because most strokes in patients randomized to warfarin occurred while the patients were not in fact taking warfarin or were significantly under-anticoagulated at the time of the event. Overall, the data from the trials suggest that treating 1,000 patients with warfarin over 12 months will prevent 30 strokes. A similar reduction in

relative risk for secondary prevention translates into the prevention of 80 strokes a year for every 1,000 patients treated. In these trials the overall incidence of haemorrhage was 1.3% a year for those receiving warfarin than 0.9% a year for the control group.

A recent small uncontrolled observational study set in secondary care, of 167 patients, of whom one half were over the age of 75 years, suggests that anticoagulation of patients not currently on treatment might result in similar rates of stroke and major haemorrhage to those achieved in the trials. The absolute benefit of warfarin depends upon balancing the underlying risk of stroke and risk of haemorrhage and this study was of insufficient size to exclude an important excess risk of haemorrhage and did not draw patients from a primary care setting.

Patients with paroxysmal AF are at similar stroke risk to patients with sustained AF. The most recent analysis from the Stroke Prevention in AF Investigators reported that 460 patients with paroxysmal AF had stroke rates and risk factors similar to patients in sustained AF, and these patients were likely to benefit from anticoagulation. Thus, patients with paroxysmal AF should be managed in a similar way to patients with sustained AF, with long-term anticoagulation for high-risk patients. If these patients are not anticoagulated when they present with an acute episode of AF, they should be managed with intravenous heparin and (if the duration of AF is >48 hours) warfarin, as described above, before cardioversion.

Atrial fibrillation patients presenting with stroke

Some patients with acute AF present with an acute stroke or thromboembolic event. A proposed management approach is summarized below, although these recommendations are not based on any randomized controlled trial evidence. Before warfarin or any antithrombotic agent is commenced, a computed tomography (CT) or MRI scan performed 48 hours or more after symptom onset should confirm the absence of intracranial haemorrhage.

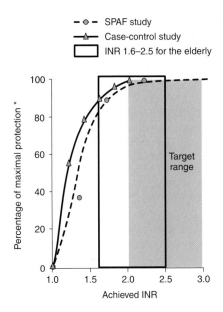

Figure 9.1
Thromboprophylaxis in atrial fibrillation: relative efficacy of target INRs of 2.0–3.0. *Presumes maximal protection with INRs >2.0. Adapted from Hart RG, Benavente O. *Proc R Coll Physicians Edinb* 1999; **29**(Suppl 3): 20–6.

The debate over the role of thrombolytic therapy for early acute ischaemic stroke is beyond the scope of this book.

Risk stratification

The risk of stroke and of thromboembolic events in AF varies widely, depending on the presence or absence of associated risk factors. Thus, risk stratification of a patient with AF is possible and is useful in assessing the risk and benefit of starting anti-thrombotic therapy. One practical risk stratification scheme based on the analyses from the AF investigators is summarized in Table 9.1. A comparison with other risk stratification criteria is shown in Table 9.2.

Stroke with intermittent atrial fibrillation: incidence and predictors during aspirin therapy
(from Hart RG, Pearce LA, Rothbart RM *et al*. J Am Coll Cardiol 2000; 35: 183–7).

The annualized rate of ischaemic stroke was similar for those with intermittent (3.2%) and sustained (3.3%) atrial fibrillation.

In patients with intermittent AF, independent predictors of stroke were:

- Advancing age (relative risk [RR] = 2.1 per decade, *p*<0.001)
- Hypertension (RR = 3.4, *p*=0.003)
- Prior stroke (RR = 4.1, *p*=0.01)
- Of those with intermittent AF, predicted to be high risk (24%), the observed stroke rate was 7.8% per year (95% CI 4.5–14)

Antithrombotic therapy in AF patients presenting with acute strokes

- Warfarin (target INR 2.0–3.0) could be commenced in non-hypertensive patients with small sized strokes.
- Anticoagulation should be postponed for one to two weeks in patients with large thromboembolic strokes due to the potential risk of haemorrhagic transformation.
- The acute use of oral aspirin in the International Stroke Trial and the Chinese Acute Stroke Trial led to a marginal benefit in mortality but this appeared to be less so among patients with AF at time of presentation, in view of the likelihood of embolization of pre-existing thrombi rather than the prevention of new thrombus formation *per se*.

Table 9.1
Risk stratification and anticoagulation in non-valvular AF (NVAF)

Assess risk:
1. **High risk** (annual risk of CVA = 8–12%)
- All patients with NVAF and previous transient ischaemic attack (TIA) or CVA
- All patients aged 75 and over with NVAF and diabetes and/or hypertension
- All patients with NVAF and clinical evidence of valve disease, heart failure, thyroid disease and/or impaired LV function on echocardiography*
2. **Moderate risk** (annual risk of CVA = 4%)
- All patients under 65 with NVAF and clinical risk factors: diabetes, hypertension, peripheral arterial disease, and ischaemic heart disease
- All patients over 65 with NVAF who have not been identified in high-risk group
3. **Low risk** (annual risk of CVA = 1%)
- All other patients under 65 with NVAF with no history of embolism, hypertension, diabetes or other clinical risk factors.

Reassess risk factors at regular intervals

Treatment:
- High risk: use warfarin (target INR 2.0–3.0) if no contraindications and possible in practice
- Moderate risk: use either warfarin or aspirin. In view of insufficient clearcut evidence, treatment may be decided on individual cases. Referral and echocardiography may help
- Low risk: use aspirin 75–300 mg daily

*Echocardiogram not needed for routine risk assessment but refines clinical risk stratification in case of impaired LV function and valve disease (see 1 above). A large left atrium *per se* is not an independent risk factor on multivariate analysis.

CVA = Cerebrovascular accident

Adapted from Lip GYH. *Lancet* 1999; **353**: 4–6.

Table 9.2
Comparison of risk stratification schemes for prevention of stroke in non-valvular AF

Criteria (year)	High risk	Intermediate risk	Low risk
Atrial Fibrillation Investigators (1994)	Age ≥ 65years History of hypertension Diabetes mellitus	Age ≥ 65years History of hypertension Diabetes mellitus	Age <65 years No high-risk features
American College of Chest Physicians Consensus (1998)	Age >75 years History of hypertension Left ventricular dysfunction# >one moderate risk factor	Age 65–75 years Diabetes mellitus Coronary disease (Thyrotoxicosis)*	Age <65 years No risk factors
Stroke Prevention in Atrial Fibrillation (1995)	Women >75 years Systolic blood pressure >160 mmHg Left ventricular dysfunction†	History of hypertension No high-risk features	No high-risk features No history of hypertension
Lip GYH (1999)	Patients ≥75 years and with diabetes or hypertension Patients with clinical evidence of heart failure, thyroid disease, and/or impaired left ventricular function on echocardiography‡	Patients <65 years with clinical risk factors: diabetes, hypertension, peripheral arterial disease, ischaemic heart disease Patients over 65 not identified in high risk group	Patients <65 years with no risk factors

*Patients with thyrotoxicosis were excluded from participation in the test cohort. #Moderate to severe left ventricular dysfunction on echocardiography. †Recent congestive heart failure or fractional shortening ≤25% by M-mode echocardiography. ‡Echocardiography not needed for routine risk assessment but refines clinical risk stratification in case of impaired left-ventricular function and valve disease.

Adapted from Pearce LA, Hart RG, Halperin JL. *Am J Med* 2000; **109**: 45–51.

A recent analysis from the SPAF Investigators of 2012 patients prescribed aspirin therapy confirmed that age, female sex, history of hypertension, systolic blood pressure >160 mmHg and prior stroke or transient ischaemic attack, as well as hormone replacement therapy (HRT) use, were independently associated with stroke risk, but not heart failure. Regular alcohol consumption reduced stroke risk. It should therefore be feasible to identify 'high risk' patients who would benefit most from anticoagulation.

The EAFT investigators conducted a similar analysis of the placebo-treated group of the EAFT secondary prevention trial, which included patients with one or more non-disabling episodes of cerebral ischaemia and AF. They found that previous thromboembolism, systolic BP >160 mmHg, duration of AF for more than one year, presence of cerebral infarct on CT scan and cardiothoracic ratio >50% on chest X-ray were significant predictors of stroke risk in multi-variate analysis. Ischaemic heart disease was a predictor of vascular events (but not stroke). A risk stratification scheme was produced whereby risk in patients with previous transient ischaemic attack (TIA) or minor stroke varied between 0% (with wide confidence intervals) and 37% per annum.

Aspirin should be administered to patients who have contraindications to warfarin therapy. Patients should be well informed about the benefits and the risks of therapy. Importantly, risk stratification for thromboprophylaxis in AF is not a static process and patients who are judged to be at low risk of stroke and are not given warfarin should be periodically re-evaluated.

Bleeding risks

Careful patient selection (assessing for bleeding risk and compliance), patient education, INR monitoring, and regular medical supervision play vital roles in reducing the bleeding risks of anticoagulation therapy for AF.

There are three issues:

- What is the risk of haemorrhage observed in the trials?

- What is the risk of haemorrhage in routine clinical practice?

- What factors increase the risk of haemorrhage in individual patients?

Rate of haemorrhage in trials

The annual risks of intracranial haemorrhage increase from 0.1% in controls to 0.3% in warfarin groups, which represents an excess of two intracranial bleeds per annum per thousand patients treated. Expressed in another way, the major bleeding rate was 1.3% per year in the warfarin group, vs. 1.0% per year in the control. The AF investigators' meta-analysis reported a rate of 1.3% per year in the warfarin group of major haemorrhage as compared to 1.0% per year in the control group (ie three extra major haemorrhages per 1000 patients per year). Major haemorrhage was defined as intracranial bleeding or a bleeding event requiring two units of blood or hospital admission. Just under one-half of the haemorrhages were intracranial or intracerebral.

The rate of minor haemorrhage from the trials has been estimated as 9.2% per annum. The one trial to report higher bleeding rates was SPAF II: 2.3% per annum on warfarin versus 1.1% per annum on aspirin, which almost offset the beneficial reduction in ischaemic stroke among the patients aged >75 years (1.8%/year) [RR 2.6, vs those aged <75]. This trial had a very wide target INR (2.0–4.5), and included a higher proportion of elderly patients; most bleeds also occurred at INR values >3.5. The rate of intracranial haemorrhage in this group was substantially higher than that reported in the original five trials (on average 0.3%/year).

Risk of haemorrhage in clinical practice

There is some evidence that similar haemorrhage rates to those observed in the trials can be achieved in clinical practice. In a prospective cohort study (ISCOAT) of 2745 patients drawn from 34 anticoagulation clinics in Italy, there were 1.3 major haemorrhages per 100 patient years (including 0.25 fatal cerebral haemorrhages) and 6.2 minor haemorrhages. Since this study included anticoagulation for all indications, the mean age of patients (62 years) was lower than would be anticipated for anticoagulation for AF.

A prospective cohort study set in the UK of anticoagulation for AF found that the incidence of major haemorrhage was 1.7% per annum and of minor haemorrhage 5.4% per annum in 167 patients with a mean age of 77 years. Higher rates of major haemorrhage were observed in a US cohort (11% per annum) that recruited patients between 1977 and 1983. The incidence of fatal haemorrhage was approximately 2% per annum. This is likely to be explained by the higher target range for anticoagulation at that time, and perhaps a different case definition of 'major' haemorrhage.

What factors increase risk of haemorrhage?

There are two approaches to ascertaining what factors are associated with increased risk of haemorrhage: cohort studies (including the treatment arms of randomized trials) and case control studies.

Cohort studies

In the Italian study mentioned above (ISCOAT) of 2745 patients (mean age 62 years, both AF and non-AF) from 34 anticoagulation clinics, there were 1.3 major haemorrhages per 100 patient years (including 0.25 fatal cerebral haemorrhages) and 6.2 minor haemorrhages. The risk was found to be higher for older patients (RR

1.75 in people aged 70 or over as compared to under 70), during the first 90 days of treatment (RR 1.75), and higher INRs. Analysis of the SPAF II study also demonstrated an association with age (RR 2.6 for patients aged over 75 years as compared to those under 75) and with intensity of anticoagulation, and found an association with the number of prescribed medications. The study of Landefeld et al identified age, history of stroke, history of gastro-intestinal bleeding, serious co-morbidity and AF as independent risk factors for haemorrhage.

One retrospective cohort study of 928 patients on warfarin in five US anticoagulation clinics also found an association with high anticoagulation, recent initiation of warfarin therapy (ie in 90 days), and the presence of three or more co-morbid conditions. Unlike the other studies, age and use of other drugs were not found to be risk factors. This perhaps reflects the young age of the study population (mean age: 57 years). A later study by the same group that included a prospective cohort, and increased the number of patients to 2376, still did not find an increased risk in association with age, except for people aged over 80. A cohort study of 6814 patients in Holland recruited during 1988 did find age and achieved intensity of anticoagulation to be important risk factors. The recent prospective cohort study by Kalra et al to determine if trial efficacy of anticoagulation for stroke prevention in AF translated into clinical effectiveness, found the incidence of major haemorrhage was 1.7% per annum and of minor haemorrhage 5.4% per annum, in 167 patients with a mean age of 77 years.

Case controlled studies

Level of anticoagulation achieved, age, history of stroke and presence of a prosthetic heart valve were identified as significant risk factors in the case control study by Hylek and Singer. A nested case control study in ISCOAT confirmed an increased risk of intra-cranial bleeding in the elderly. In the ISCOAT study, the relative risk was 1.75 in people aged ≥70 years compared to

those <70 years, during the first 90 days of treatment (RR 1.75) and higher INRs.

Increased bleeding risk with anticoagulation in AF

Associated with the following features:
- An INR greater than 3.0
- Fluctuating INRs
- Uncontrolled hypertension
- Age >75 years

Even low-dose aspirin increases the risk of major haemorrhage by two-fold (0.5% per year in elderly people). One meta-analysis of 16 randomized trials involving aspirin use, with 55,462 participants, estimated an excess risk of haemorrhagic stroke or 1.2 per 1000 patient years. The adverse effects of aspirin on the gastrointestinal tract, which are often dose-related, could vary from dyspepsia to life threatening haemorrhage.

Other strategies in providing thromboprophylaxis

One possible strategy in providing thromboprophylaxis is the use of new antiplatelet agents, or combination therapy of agents that inhibit the platelet via different pathways.

For example, the SIFA (Studio Italiano Fibrillazione Atriale) study compared the efficacy of indobufen, a new antiplatelet agent, against warfarin in secondary prevention of stroke in 916 patients with AF and a recent cerebral ischaemic episode who were randomized to indobufen or warfarin (target INR 2.0–3.5). In SIFA, there was no significant difference in the primary event rate in the two groups (10% per annum in the warfarin group; 12% in the indobufen group), with a reduced bleeding risk in the indobufen group. The primary endpoint for this trial was the combined incidence of stroke (including haemorrhagic), pulmonary or systemic embolus, non-fatal myocardial infarction and vascular death.

In the second European Stroke Prevention Study (ESPS-2), which was a secondary prevention study, low-dose aspirin (50 mg) alone, sustained release dipyridamole (400 mg/day) alone, or a combination of the two agents, were compared with placebo over 24 months. This study found that dipyridamole reduced the risk of stroke by 22% relative to placebo, while the combination of dipyridamole and aspirin reduced the risk of stroke by 43% relative to placebo; indeed, combination therapy was superior to either agent alone in preventing stroke. Although only a small proportion of patients in ESPS-2 had AF, a post-hoc subgroup analysis suggested non-significant trends towards benefits in patients with AF taking aspirin–dipyridamole combination therapy.

Treatment regimes using low-intensity warfarin–aspirin combination therapy and fixed dose warfarin were tested in a series of randomized trials conducted in the 1990s, which compared fixed low-dose warfarin regimes (eg warfarin 1.25 mg), or low-intensity warfarin (INR <1.5) in combination with aspirin, as alternatives to conventional anticoagulation (INR 2.0–3.0) or aspirin in patients with AF. Nevertheless the results from these trials were disappointing, and such regimes should not be used as thromboprophylaxis in AF.

Do the anticoagulation trials represent clinical practice?

- Trials have carefully selected patient populations.
- Anticoagulation was strictly monitored by well-motivated investigators in trial populations.
- Trial patients essentially received careful follow-up and 'packages of care'.

Whether or not the results from AF anticoagulation trials could be fully extrapolated to general clinical practice is not entirely clear.

From trials to clinical practice

Care should be employed when interpreting the results of the clinical trials, which demonstrate unequivocal benefit of anticoagulation in AF. While efforts have been made at attaining optimal management of anticoagulation as shown in the trials, many of the observational studies in the UK indicate that there is considerable variation in the antithrombotic management of AF and still a considerable proportion of eligible patients are not adequately managed. Until we can develop more effective, efficient and safe methods of providing adequate thromboprophylaxis, efforts at careful risk stratification with clinical risk factors (with some refinement from echocardiography) are needed.

Contraindications to warfarin

The patient:
- Co-morbidity – medical conditions, falls, frailty, exposure to trauma, etc.
- Cognitive function
- ?Housebound

The doctor:
- Drug interactions
- Organization of INR monitoring

The system:
- GP vs hospital facilities, eg remote location
- Resources

Initiating warfarin

The 'Fennerty regime' comprises warfarin 10 mg on day one, with subsequent doses tailored to INR measurements. Modifications been made particularly for elderly patients, with warfarin 5 mg daily for four days, followed by subsequent doses defined by a nomogram.

Anticoagulation monitoring

Traditionally, measurement of patient's anticoagulation was in busy, congested, hospital-based clinics. This is despite some evidence that more efficient anticoagulation control is achieved if general practitioners undertake anticoagulation monitoring. Computerized programmes (referred to as 'computerized decision support systems' [CDSS]) have been developed to manage anticoagulation dosing, the reliability of which appear to be either as good as or better than warfarin dosing by experienced medical staff. Self-testing and even self-management of anticoagulation intensity by the patient results in as good or even better control of anticoagulation than physician-managed anticoagulation, and may become widespread practice in the future, especially with increasing numbers of patients taking anticoagulant therapy for conditions such as AF.

Delivery of anticoagulation therapy

- Anticoagulant clinics
  - Busy/congested
  - Increasing problem, especially with more elderly population
  - Inconvenient
- Domicillary anticoagulation service
  - Resources
  - Limited availability
  - Immobile, housebound, etc.
- 'Near-patient' testing
  - Resources
  - Dependent on primary care/facilities/ training

Further reading

Albers G, Dalen J, Laupacis A et al. Antithrombotic therapy in atrial fibrillation. Chest 2001; **119**: 194S–206S.

Atrial Fibrillation Investigators. The efficacy of aspirin in patients with atrial fibrillation. Analysis of pooled data from three randomized trials. Arch Intern Med 1997; **157**: 1237–40.

Atrial fibrillation investigators. Risk factors for stroke and efficacy of antithrombotic therapy in atrial fibrillation. Analysis of pooled data from five randomised controlled trials. Arch Intern Med 1994; **154**: 1449–57.

Benavente O, Hart R, Koudstaal P et al. Oral anticoagulants for preventing stroke in patients with non-valvular atrial fibrillation and no previous history of stroke or transient ischaemic attack (Cochrane Review). In: The Cochrane Library, Issue 1, 2000.

CAST: randomised placebo-controlled trial of early aspirin use in 20,000 patients with acute ischaemic stroke. CAST (Chinese Acute Stroke Trial) Collaborative Group. Lancet 1997; **349**: 1641–9.

Diener HC, Cunha L, Forbes C et al. European Stroke Prevention Study. 2. Dipyridamole and acetylsalicylic acid in the secondary prevention of stroke. J Neurol Sci 1996; **143**: 1–13.

Ezekowitz MD, Levine JA. Preventing stroke in patients with atrial fibrillation. JAMA 1999; **281**(19): 1830–5.

Fennerty J et al. Flexible induction dose regimen for warfarin and prediction of maintenance dose. BMJ 1984; **288**: 1268–70.

Fihn SD, McDonell M, Martin D et al. Risk factors for complications of chronic anticoagulation: a multicentre study. Ann Intern Med 1993; **118**: 511–20.

Fihn SD, Calahan CM, Martin DC et al. The risk for and severity of bleeding complications in elderly patients treated with warfarin. Ann Intern Med 1996; **124**: 970–9.

Gullov AL, Koefoed BG, Petersen P et al. Fixed minidose warfarin and aspirin alone and in combination vs adjusted dose warfarin for stroke prevention in atrial fibrillation. Arch Intern Med. 1998; **158**: 1513–21.

Hart RG et al. Factors associated with ischaemic stroke during aspirin therapy in AF: analysis of 2,012 participants in the SPAF I-III clinical trials. Stroke 1999; **30**: 1223–9.

Hart RG, Pearce LA, Rothbart RM et al. Stroke with intermittent atrial fibrillation: incidence and predictors during aspirin therapy. J Am Coll Cardiol 2000; **35**: 183–7.

Hart RG. Antithrombotic therapy to prevent stroke in patients with AF: a meta-analysis. Ann Intern Med 1999; **131**: 492–500.

He J, Whelton P K, Vu B, Klag M J. Aspirin and risk of hemorrhagic stroke: a meta-analysis of RCTs. JAMA 1998; **280**(22): 1930–5.

Hellemons BSP, Langenberg M, Lodder J et al. Primary prevention of arterial thromboembolism in non-rheumatic atrial fibrillation in primary care: RCT comparing two intensities of coumarin with aspirin. BMJ 1999; **319**: 958–64.

Hylek EM, Singer DE. Risk factors for intracranial haemorrhage in outpatients taking warfarin. Ann Intern Med 1994; **120**: 897–902.

Hylek EM, Skates SJ, Sheehan MA et al. An analysis of the lowest effective intensity of prophylactic anticoagulation for patients with nonrheumatic atrial fibrillation. N Engl J Med 1996; **335**: 540–6.

Kalra L et al. Prospective cohort study to determine if trial efficacy of anticoagulation for stroke prevention in atrial fibrillation translates into clinical effectiveness. BMJ 2000; **320**: 1236–9.

Klein AL, Grimm RA, Black IW et al. Cardioversion guided by transesophageal echocardiography: the ACUTE Pilot Study. A randomized, controlled trial. Assessment of

Cardioversion Using Transesophageal Echocardiography. *Ann Intern Med* 1997; **126**: 200–9.

Koudstaal P. Anticoagulants for preventing stroke in patients with nonrheumatic atrial fibrillation and a history of stroke or transient ischemic attacks (Cochrane Review). In: The Cochrane Library, Issue 1, 2000. Oxford: Update Software.

Landefeld CS, Goldman L. Major bleeding in outpatients treated with warfarin: incidence and prediction by factors known at the start of outpatient therapy. *Am J Med* 1989; **87**: 145–52.

Lin HJ, Wolf PA, Kelly-Hayes M *et al*. Stroke severity in atrial fibrillation. The Framingham Study. *Stroke* 1996; **27**: 1760–4.

Lip GYH. Does paroxysmal atrial fibrillation confer a paroxysmal thromboembolic risk? *Lancet* 1997; **349**: 1565–6.

Lip GYH. Thromboprophylaxis for atrial fibrillation. *Lancet* 1999; **353**: 4–6.

Morocutti C, Amabile G, Fattapposta F *et al*. Indobufen versus warfarin in the secondary prevention of major vascular events in nonrheumatic atrial fibrillation. SIFA (Studio Italiano Fibrillazione Atriale) investigators. *Stroke* 1997; **28**: 1015–21.

Palareti G, Leali N, Coccheri S *et al*. Bleeding complications of oral anticoagulant treatment: an inception cohort, prospective collaborative study (ISCOAT). *Lancet* 1996; **348**: 423–8.

Palaretti G, Hirsh J, Legnani C *et al*. Oral anticoagulation treatment in the elderly: a nested prospective case control study. *Arch Intern Med* 2000; **160**: 470–8.

Pell JP, McIver B, Stuart P *et al*. Comparison of anticoagulant control among patients attending general practice and a hospital anticoagulant clinic. *Br J Gen Prac* 1993; **43**: 152–4.

SPAF Investigators. Bleeding during antithrombotic therapy in patients with atrial fibrillation. *Arch Intern Med* 1996; **156**: 409–16.

Stroke Prevention in Atrial Fibrillation Investigators. Warfarin versus aspirin for prevention of thromboembolism in atrial fibrillation: Stroke Prevention in Atrial Fibrillation II Study. *Lancet* 1994; **343**: 687–91.

The International Stroke Trial (IST): a randomised trial of aspirin, subcutaneous heparin, both, or neither among 19,435 patients with acute ischaemic stroke. International Stroke Trial Collaborative Group. *Lancet* 1997; **349**: 1569–81.

van der Meer FJM, Rosendaal FR, Vandenbroucke JP *et al*. Bleeding complications in oral anticoagulant therapy: an analysis of risk factors. *Arch Intern Med* 1993; **153**: 1557–62.

van Latum JC *et al* for the EAFT Study Group. Predictors of major vascular events in patients with a TIA or minor ischaemic stroke and with NRAF. *Stroke* 1995; **26**: 801–6.

Index

Page numbers in *italics* refer to information that is shown only in a table or figure

Note: atrial fibrillation is abbreviated to AF